Basic Principles of Chromatography & HPLC

Basic Principles of Chromatography & HPLC

Arunadevi S. Birajdar

Associate Professor
*K.T. Patil College of Pharmacy,
Osmanabad Maharashtra*

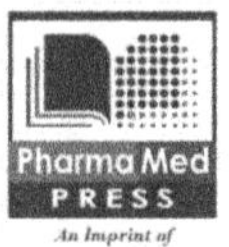

PharmaMed Press

An imprint of BSP Books Pvt. Ltd

4-4-309/316, Giriraj Lane,
Sultan Bazar, Hyderabad - 500 095.

Published by:

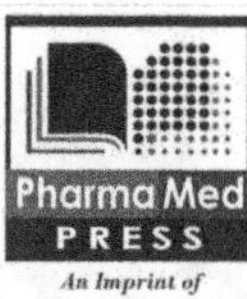

PharmaMed Press

An imprint of BSP Books Pvt. Ltd.

4-4-309/316, Giriraj Lane, Sultan Bazar, Hyderabad - 500 095.

Phone: 040-23445688; Fax: 91+40-23445611

e-mail: info@pharmamedpress.com

www.pharmamedpress.com/www.pharmamedpress.net

ISBN: 978-93-95039-08-6 (Hardback)

Preface

This book is a self explanatory book to understanding the basics of chromatography. I have tried to share my knowledge and put together a complete theoretical and practical approach to one instrumental technique, HPLC, in simple English. HPLC is an essential instrument used for the separation and analysis of chemicals as well as drug molecules. It is the most important method of analysis and is helpful for the study of organic and inorganic compound analysis. The aim of this book's publication is to create an interest in students to study and understand pharmaceutical analysis by HPLC in detail and to provide an introduction to UPLC. This book can be used by UG as well as PG students of pharmacy and analytical chemistry to learn the basics of HPLC method development and the estimation of drugs using this instrument. The essentials of new method development, validation in accordance with ICH guidelines, and calibration techniques are also thoroughly explained.

It's my pleasure to write this book to support the teaching staff and students in gaining insights and knowledge on this subject. I am thankful to my management, staff, and my brothers for their support in writing this small textbook.

- Author

Contents

Chapter – 7

High-Performance Liquid Chromatography (HPLC)

Chapter – 8

Detail Instrumentation of HPLC

Chapter – 9

Types of Elution

Chapter – 10

Calibration and Validation (HPLC)

Chapter – 11

New Method Development & Validation as per ICH Guidelines

Chapter – 12

Validation of New HPLC Method Developed as per ICH Guidelines

Chapter – 13

Applications of Column Chromatograpy and HPLC

Chapter – 14

Ultra High-Performance Liquid Chromatography (UPLC) Or (UHPLC)

INTRODUCTION TO CHROMATOGRAPHY

Drug analysis, namely, identification, characterization and determination of drugs in dosage forms and biological fluids, play an important role in the development, manufacture and therapeutic use of the drug. Drugs are developed and manufactured as dosage form prior to their use by patients. Dosage forms require a variety of tests and standards to assure their therapeutic benefits. Administration of two or more drugs at a time becomes necessary for several therapeutic reasons. There exist several drug combinations, referred to as multi-component dosage forms, which have proved to be effective due to their combined mode of action in the body. These drug combinations not only offer better therapeutically effective due to additive or synergistic effects but are also administrated as a single dosage, economy in production.

This book deals with the studies carried out by the writer in her teaching experience for the past Twenty Six years in the Pharmaceutical Analysis subject and Research carried out on the development and validation of HPLC and spectrophotometric methods for selected multi-component drugs in their formulations.

IMPORTANCE OF NEWER ANALYTICAL METHODS

The number of drugs and drug formulations introduced into the market by pharmaceutical industries has been increasing at an alarming rate. These drugs or formulations may be either new entities or partial structural modifications of the existing ones or novel dosage forms (controlled/ sustained release formulations), or multi-component dosage forms.

The development of newer analytical methods for the estimation of these drugs or drug combinations is necessary because of the following reasons:

- Analytical methods for the quantification of the drugs in different combination forms and biological fluids may not be available.
- The drug combination may not be official in any pharmacopoeia
- A literature search may not reveal any analytical procedure and methods for drug combinations due to the interference caused by excipients
- Analytical methods for a drug in combination with other drugs may not be available

Newer methods are also recommended when the existing methods,

- May require expensive instruments, reagents and solvents used,
- May involve cumbersome extraction or separation steps which are time-consuming and
- May not be simple, rapid, reliable and sensitive.

ESTIMATION OF DRUGS IN THEIR FORMULATIONS

Estimation of drugs in their formulations, however, is difficult because of the presence of one or more drug components in addition to additives. In the process of estimation, it is important to confirm that one component does not interfere with the estimation of the other. The complexity of these formulations thus poses a challenge to the analytical chemist during the development of dosage form assay methods. Analytical methods for the estimation of drugs in their formulations include:

1. Classical separation and analysis

The components of interest are subjected to classical separation techniques like extraction or isolation in this process. A suitable estimation procedure is then selected to quantify the components by gravimetric and volumetric methods.

(a) Volumetric Analysis (Different types of Titrations)

(b) Gravimetric Analysis (Precipitation Analysis)

2. Spectral methods

Spectral techniques are used to measure the electromagnetic radiation, which is either absorbed or emitted by the sample as a function of the drug concentration, UV-Visible spectroscopy, fluorimetry, flame photometry, and NMR are some of the important techniques.

3. Electroanalytical methods

They involve the measurement of current, voltage or resistance as a property of the concentration of the drug component. Potentiometer, Conductometry and Amperometry are some of the important techniques.

4. Chromatographic methods

Chromatography is a method of separation where the individual components are separated and analyzed. In this technique, two or more components are separated by a dynamic differential migration process in a system consisting of two phases, one of which moves continuously in a given direction in which the individual components exhibit different mobility due to the difference in their adsorption or partition or molecular size etc. The most reliable and widely used chromatographic techniques used for the estimation of drugs in their formulations are

(a) Gas-liquid chromatography (GLC)

In this technique, a carrier gas is used as the mobile phase that passes over a liquid non-volatile stationary phase, coated on an inert solid support. The separation is effected in accordance with the difference in partition coefficients of the components.

(b) High-performance thin-layer chromatography (HPTLC)

This is a sophisticated, advanced and automated version of thin-layer chromatography. It is the fastest-growing technique for the analysis of drugs.

(c) High-performance liquid chromatography (HPLC)

HPLC is a type of chromatography that employs a liquid mobile phase and a very finely divided stationary phase. In order to obtain satisfactory flow rates, the liquid must be pressurized to several hundred pounds per square inch or more. The high-performance liquid chromatography technique is so called because of its improved performance compared to classical column chromatography.

BASIC CLASSIFICATION & THEORY OF CHROMATOGRAPHY

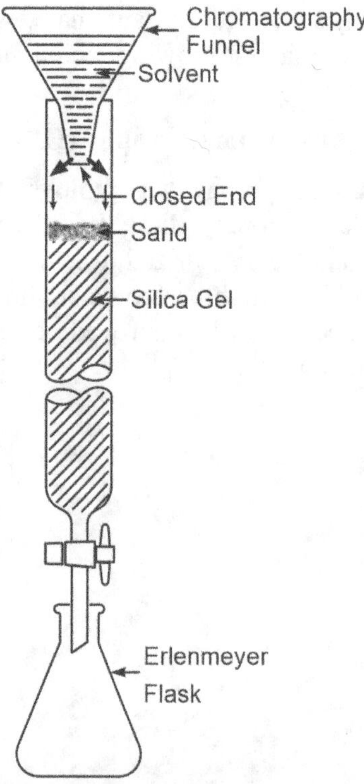

Fig. 2.1 Column Chromatography.

A technique for analysis of chemical substances. The term *chromatography* literally means colour writing, and denotes a method by which the substance to be analysed is poured into a vertical glass tube containing an adsorbent, the various components of the substance moving through the adsorbent at different rates, according to their degree of attraction to it, and producing bands of colour at different levels of the adsorption column. The term has been extended to include other methods utilising the same principle, although no colours are produced in the column.

The mobile phase of chromatography refers to the fluid that carries the mixture of substances in the sample through the adsorptive material. The stationary phase (or adsorbent) refers to the solid material that takes up the particles of the substance passing through it. Kaolin, alumina, silica and activated charcoal have been used as adsorbing substances or stationary phases.

Classification of chromatographic techniques tends to be confusing because it may be based on the type of stationary phase, the nature of the adsorptive force, the nature of the mobile phase, or the method by which the mobile phase is introduced.

The technique is a valuable tool for the research biochemist and is readily adaptable to investigations conducted in the clinical laboratory. For example, chromatography is used to detect and identify in body fluids certain sugars and amino acids associated with inborn errors of metabolism.

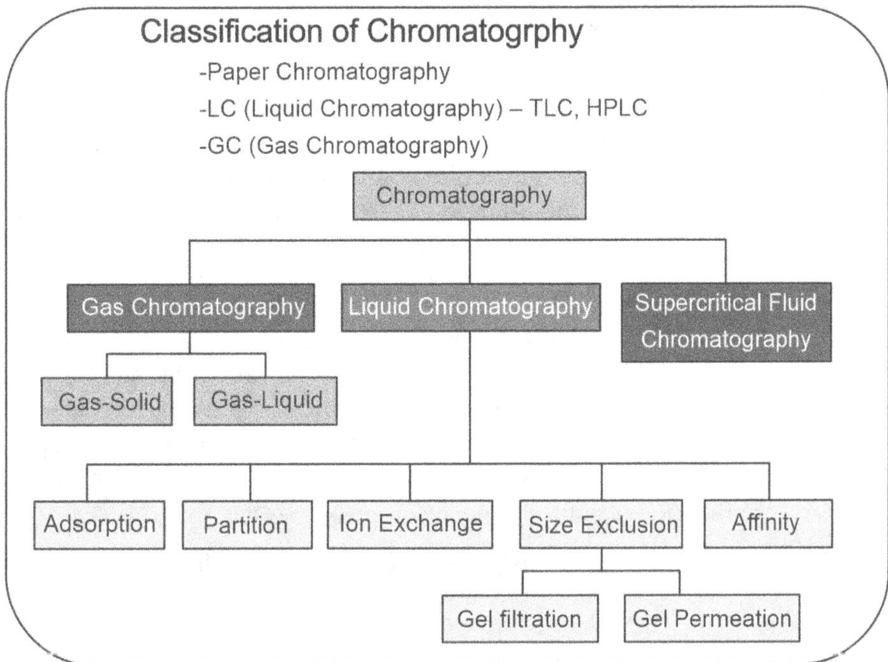

Fig. 2.2 The Classification of Chromatography Systems.

(a) Adsorption chromatography

That is a technique in which the stationary phase is an adsorbent. It may be solid or liquid

And separation depends on the adsorption phenomenon.

(b) Column chromatography

The technique in which the various solutes of a solution are allowed to travel down a column, the individual components being adsorbed by the stationary phase. The most strongly adsorbed component will remain near the top of the column; the other components will pass to positions farther and farther down the column according to their affinity for the adsorbent. If the individual components are naturally coloured, they will form a series of coloured bands or zones.

Column chromatography has been employed to separate vitamins, steroids, hormones and alkaloids and to determine the amount of these substances in samples of body fluids.

(c) Affinity chromatography

A method of chromatography that utilises the biologically important binding interactions that occur on protein surfaces. For example, an enzyme substrate is covalently coupled to an inert matrix such as a polysaccharide bead. The enzyme can be bound to the bead and thereby separated when present in very low concentration in a very complex mixture of other macromolecules.

(d) Size Exclusion chromatography

In which the stationary phase is a gel having a closely controlled pore size. Molecules are separated based on molecular size and shape, smaller molecules being temporarily retained in the pores.

(e) Gel-filtration chromatography, Gel-permeation chromatography

Size Exclusion chromatography.

(f) Molecular sieve chromatography

(g) Gas chromatography (GC)

A type of chromatography in which the mobile phase is an inert gas. Volatile components of the sample are separated in the column and measured by a detector. The method has been applied in the clinical laboratory to separate and quantify steroids, barbiturates and lipids.

(h) Gas-liquid chromatography (GLC)

An inert gas moves gas chromatography in which the substances are to be separated along a tube filled with a finely divided inert solid coated with a nonvolatile substance; each component migrates at a rate determined by its solubility in the stationary phase and its vapour pressure.

(i) High-performance liquid chromatography (HPLC)

A miniaturised method in which the solution to be analysed is passed, under high pressure, through a long, thin column packed with tiny beads such that analyses are completed in minutes rather than hours and with improved resolution.

(j) Ion-exchange chromatography

That utilising resins to which are coupled either cations or anions that will exchange with other cations or anions in the material passed through their meshwork.

(k) Partition chromatography

A form of separation of solutes utilises the partition of the solutes between two liquid phases, namely the original solvent and the solvent film on the adsorption column.

(l) Paper chromatography

A form of chromatography in which a sheet of special paper is substituted for the adsorption column. After separation of the components as a consequence of their differential migratory velocities, they are stained to make the chromatogram visible. In the clinical laboratory paper, chromatography is employed to detect and identify sugars and amino acids.

(m) Thin-layer chromatography

In which the stationary phase is a thin layer of an adsorbent such as silica gel coated on a flat plate. It is otherwise similar to paper chromatography.

(n) Gas-Liquid Chromatography

Gas-liquid chromatography (GC) was invented by James and Martin and is a chromatography separation technique in which the mobile phase is a gas (usually helium or nitrogen), and the stationary phase is a liquid. In the original columns used by James and Martin, the liquid stationary phase was adsorbed on the surface of inert support such as Celite (a diatomateous earth) or calcined Celite (a form of brick dust). The support was usually deactivated before use by acid treatment and subsequent reaction with hexamethyldisilazane. The technique was extensively used to separate a wide range of volatile substances. However, the packed column had a high flow impedance, which limited the column length that could be used and, consequently, the column efficiency and the resolution that could be obtained. The packed columns were eventually replaced by the capillary columns in which the mobile phase was coated on the walls of an open tube. The tubes could be 50-500 micron ID and from 10 m to several 100 m long. Thus, very fast or very efficient columns could be employed. Gas-liquid chromatography is now a very popular technique used by almost every analytical laboratory.

The primary classification of chromatography is based on the physical nature of the mobile phase. The mobile phase can be a gas or a liquid, giving rise to the two basic forms of chromatography, namely, gas chromatography (GC) and liquid chromatography (LC). The stationary phase can also take two forms, solid and liquid, which provides two subgroups of GC and LC, namely, gas-solid chromatography (GSC) and gas? Liquid chromatography (GLC), together with liquid-solid chromatography (LSC) and liquid chromatography (LLC). The different forms of chromatography are summarised in Fig.no.2.2. Most thin layer chromatography techniques are considered liquid-solid systems, although the solute normally interacts with a liquid-like surface coating on the adsorbent or support or, in some cases, an actual liquid coating. Fig no.2 The Classification of Chromatography Systems.

THEORETICAL PRINCIPLES OF CHROMATOGRAPHY

Chromatographic Process- basic Concepts

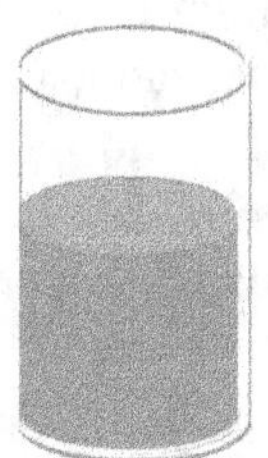

Fig 2.3 Basic separation process of Compounds in Column.

Chromatographic separation is when the analyte (sample mixture) is distributed between two phases – stationary and mobile phase. In thin-layer chromatography (TLC), the stationary phase is a plate coated with a, for example, silica gel or alumina; in HPLC, a stationary phase is a column packed with porous, surface-active particles. For TLC and HPLC, the mobile phase is liquid. In gas-liquid chromatography (GLC), the stationary phase is a thin film of liquid coated on a solid support, and the mobile phase is a gas (helium nitrogen).

The basis of the chromatographic resolution of sample mixture is the differential migration which results from the equilibrium distribution of sample components between stationary and mobile phases as shown for compounds A (Red) and B (Green) in column chromatography as shown in the below figure 2.3

Where Am & Bm are the concentration of compounds A and B in the mobile phase and As & Bs are their respective concentration in the stationary phase. S is solvent molecules of the moving phase.

The phase preference of compound A, for example, can be expressed by the distribution coefficient K, or capacity factor or capacity ratio K' is given by

$$K_p = C_{state}/C_{mob}$$

here C_{state} is the concentration of compound A in the stationary phase and C_{mob} is the concentration of compound A in the mobile phase.

$$K' = N_{state}/N_{mob}$$

Where N_{state} and N_{mob} are the number of moles of A in stationary and mobile phases, respectively. The components present in the sample mixture must have different distribution constants or capacity factors if the mixture is to be separated.

In HPLC, the sample to be analysed is injected on top of the column, and the mobile phase is pumped at a set flow rate under pressure. As the sample molecule moves along the column, spreading occurs as the compounds are eluted as Gaussian or near Gaussian peaks. This spreading or band broadening in LC is caused by rate or physical processes. These processes are

Eddy Diffusion

Eddy diffusion arises from the different solvent flow streams within the column. As a result, sample molecules take different paths through the packed column bed depending on which flow streams they follow, as shown in fig. 2.4.

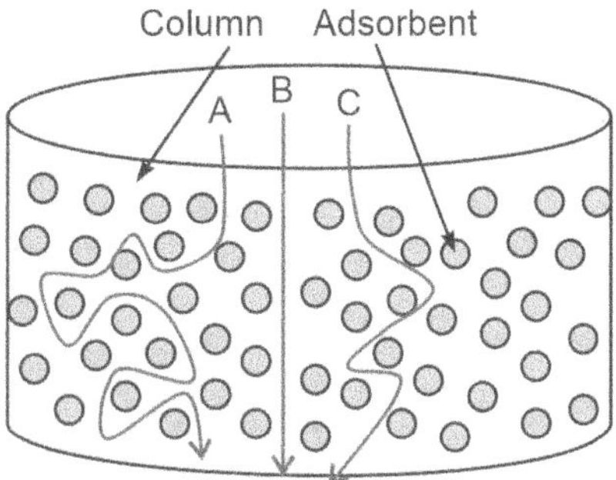

Fig. 2.4 Process of Eddy Diffusion.

Mobile Phase Mass Transfer

The mobile phase flow between the stationary phase particles is laminar, as shown in fig. 2.5. the liquid adjacent to a particle moves slower than the liquid in the centre of a flowing stream.

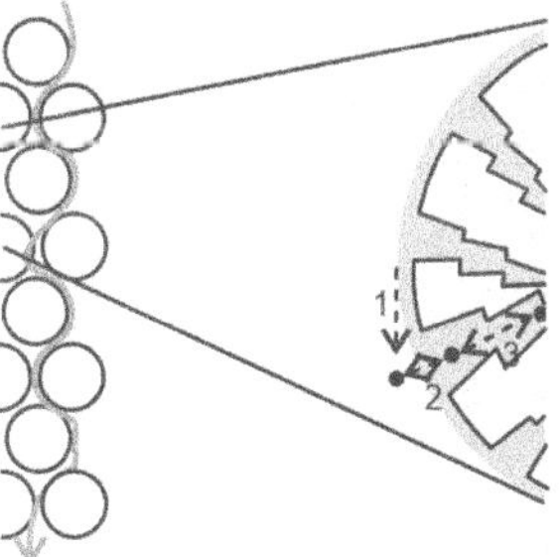

Fig 2.5 Process of Mass transfer.

Sample Molecule Diffusion in the Mobile Phase

As a result of mobile phase mass transfer, at any given time, sample molecules near the particle move a shorter distance than those in the middle of the flow stream.

Stagnant Mobile Phase Transfer

In the case of porous stationary packing particles (Fig. 2.5), the mobile phase contained within the pores of a particle is stagnant. Sample molecules that penetrate further into the pore spend more time in the pore and lower time in the external moving phase.

Longitudinal Molecular Diffusion

This effect refers to the tendency of individual molecules to diffuse randomly along the column away from the band centre.

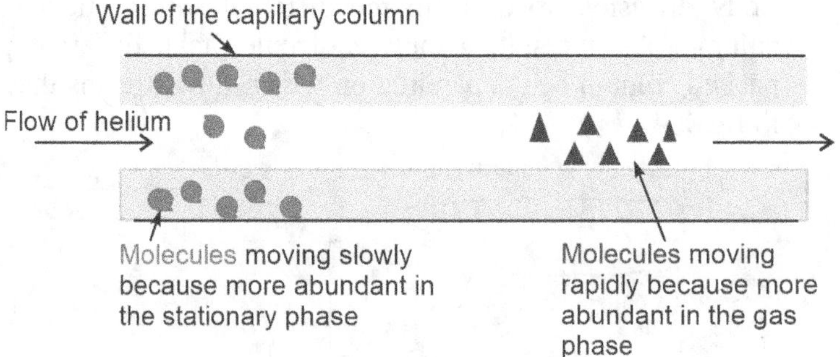

Fig. 2.6 Longitudinal Molecular diffusion.

Theoretical Plates

All factors which contribute to the peak broadening and hence to the bandwidth (tw) reduce the efficiency of an HPLC column. The bandwidth is commonly expressed in terms of the theoretical plate number N of the column and is given by

$$N == 16 \{tr/tw\}^2$$

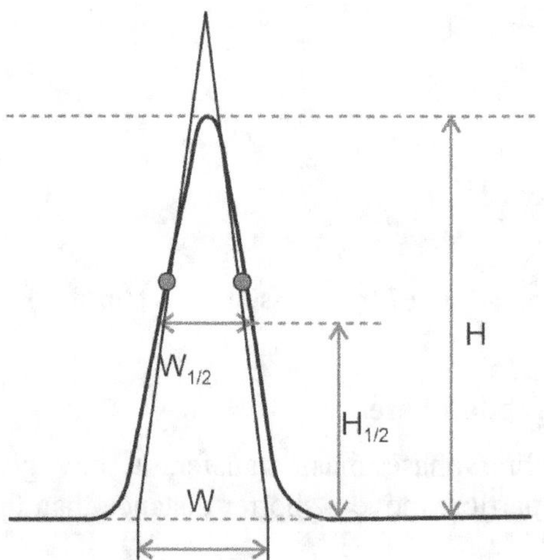

Fig. 2.7 Peak Width and Height.

Where tr and tw are the retention time and peak width of a given peak. (See fig. 2.7)

N is a useful measure of column efficiency, the relative ability of a column to give narrow peaks (Small value of tw) and improved separations.

N is proportional to column Length as N==L/H

CHROMATOGRAPHIC COLUMN EFFICIENCY IS DETERMINED BY

1- Plate height (Height Equivarent to Theoretical Plate (HETP)= L/N

2- Number of Theoretical Plates (N) =16 $(t_R/t_W)^2$

Where Wx = the width at one-twentieth of the peak height and

A = the distance between the perpendicular dropped from the peak maximum and the leading edge of the peak at one-twentieth of the peak height.

The Indian Pharmacopoeia (1996) defines column efficiency as stated in the monograph in terms of the number of the theoretical plates per meter n as follow

$$n = 5.54 V^2_R / LWh^2$$

where V_R = distance along the baseline between the point of injection and the perpendicular dropped from the maximum of the peak of interest.

L = length of the column in meters

Wh = width of the peak of interest at half peak height measured in the same unit as Vr

Where L is the column length. The proportionality constant H is the so-called height equivalent to the theoretical plate or HETP, it measures the efficiency of the column per unit length. Therefore, a small H value means a more efficient column and a large N value. A central goal in HPLC practice was and continues to be the attainment of small H values and maximum N values.

The dependence of H values as a function of all experimental conditions is described by the Van Deemter equation as follows;

$$H = A + B/u + Cu$$

Where u is the mobile phase linear velocity, A, B, and C are constants that vary from one column to another and depend to some extent on parameters such as separation temperature, mobile phase, and the analyte. A typical plot of H versus u for a column packed with less than 10 um particle size is shown in fig. 2.8.

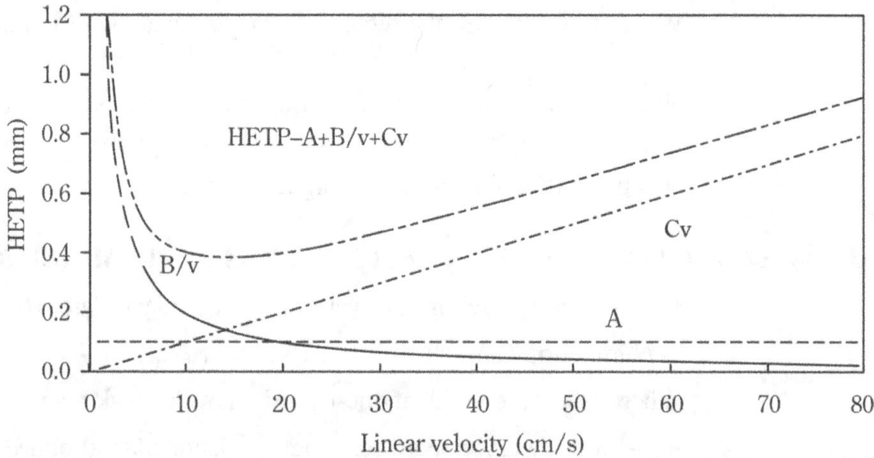

Fig. 2.8 A typical plot of H versus velocity of molecules in the column.

This is an optimum flow rate (u) for which H is a minimum and N is the maximum. HPLC columns packed with a particle size of < 10 um are usually operated at a flow rate higher than the optima to reduce analysis time.

Van deemter plots can be used as a diagnostic test to check the efficiency of the column. For each new column, Van deemter plots can be constructed as a reference point against which the column can be compared if the column efficiency deteriorates overuse. However, usually, the efficiency of the column is checked by analysing a test mixture and chromatographic conditions supplied by the column manufacturer.

The values of H for a given column are the result of not only the various band broadening processes outlined above but also contributions from plumbed components outside the column. Therefore the total peak variance (σ^2 total) arising from band broadening in a packed column is given by

$$\sigma^2{}_{total} = \sigma^2{}_{column} + \sigma^2{}_{extra\ column}$$

$$\sigma^2{}_{column} = \sigma^2{}_{d} + \sigma^2{}_{sm} + \sigma^2{}_{s} + \sigma^2{}_{e} + \sigma^2{}_{m}$$

where the terms on the right hand side of the equation corresponding to the contribution from longitudinal diffusion (d), stagnant mobile phase mass transfer (sm), stationary phase mass transfer (m), eddy diffusion (e), and mobile phase mass transfer (m) respectively.

$$\sigma^2{}_{extra\ column} = \sigma^2{}_{inj} + \sigma^2{}_{det} + \sigma^2{}_{tube}$$

Where $\sigma^2{}_{inj}$ is peak spreading contribution from the injector, $\sigma^2{}_{det}$ from the detector, $\sigma^2{}_{tub}$ from connecting tubing. The extra column contribution to peak broadening in HPLC is kept to a minimum by using good quality zero dead volume (ZDV) connectors and keeping the connecting tube as short as possible. The tubing connecting various components of the HPLC set-up is also kept of as narrow an internal diameter as possible.

There are several alternatives for calculating N, the number of theoretical plate count as shown in fig 2.9.

THE IMPORTANCE OF THEORETICAL PLATES (N)

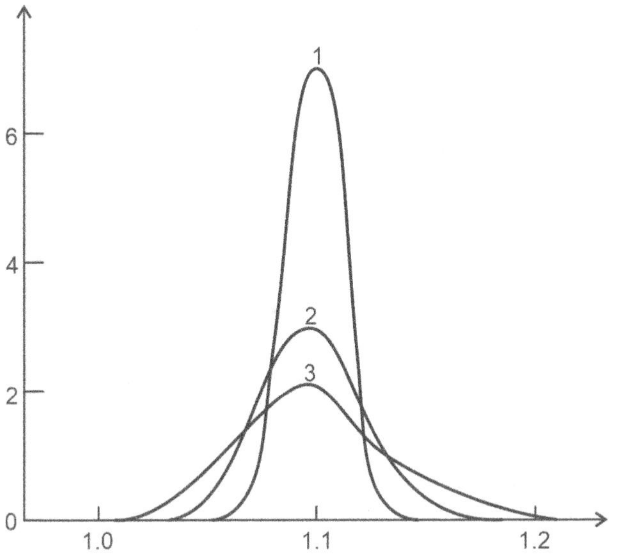

Fig.   2.9   Effect   of Bandwidth   on   Theoretical Plates.

As shown in the above figure, the relation between band width and Theoretical plates, i.e. Band Width, is directly proportional to the N number of Theoretical plates.

Peak No 1 Therotical plates 10000

Peak No 2 Therotical plates 1000

Peak No 3 Therotical plates 100

Table 2.1 Alternatives for calculation of column efficiency N

$$N = \sigma\,(VR/W)2$$

W	σ	Method
Wi	4	Inflection
Wh	5.54	½ Peak height
W3 σ	9	3 σ
Wasy	10	Asymmetry method
Ws σ	25	5 σ
Wtan	16	Tangent

The calculation of theoretical plates N, described above, assumes the peaks to be Gaussian, but in reality, chromatographic peaks are often asymmetric.

The asymmetry factor (AF) is defined as

$$A = b/a$$

Where b and a are the distances from the peak maxima of the trailing edge of the peak of interest at 5% (0.05h), 10% (0.1h) or 20% (0.2h) peak height (See Fig. 2.10)

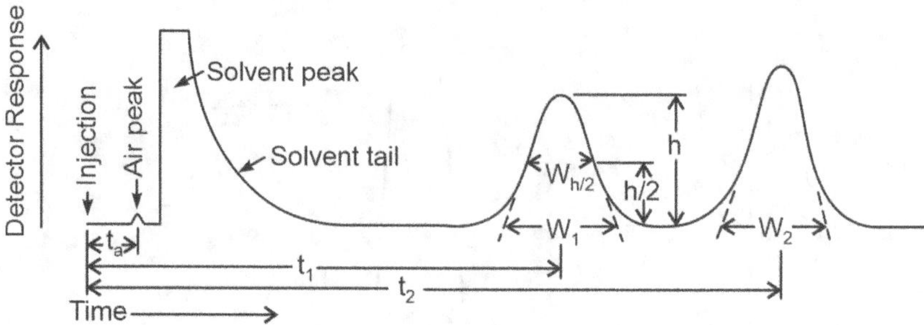

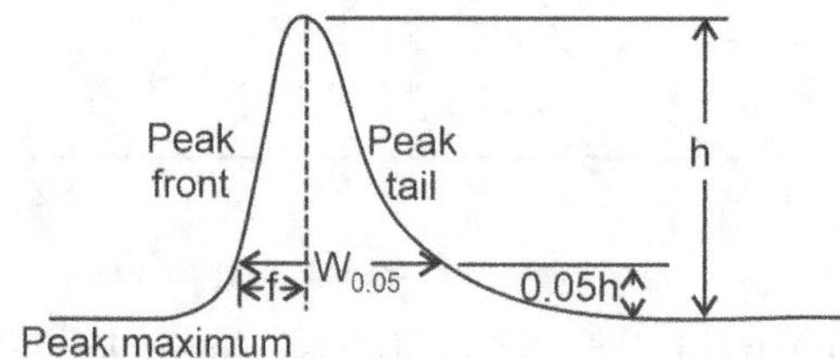

Fig. 2.10 Chromatographic separation & Asymmetric peak.

The Indian Pharmacopoeia (1996) calculates the symmetry factor of a peak from the expression.

$$Wx/2A$$

Resolution

As shown in Figures 2.10 & 2.11in a chromatogram, the quality of separation of two adjacent peaks is measured by the resolution Rs. Rs can be expressed in terms of three parameters N, α,& K', which are related to the experimental conditions as follows.

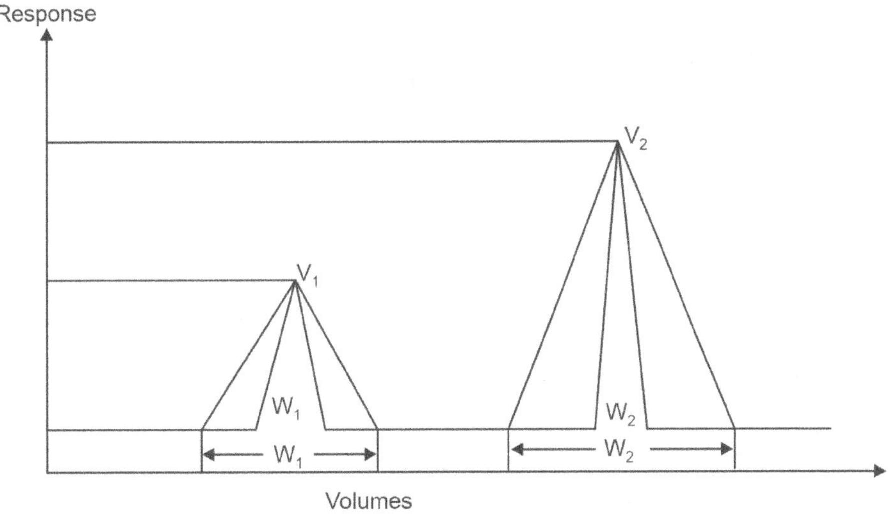

Fig. 2.11 Resolution of two peaks, V1 and V2.

Equation

Rs according to IP (1996) is given by

$$R = \frac{V_2 - V_1}{1/2(W_1 + W_2)}$$

OR

Resolution of the column (Rs) = $(V_1 - V_2)/0.5\ (W_1 + W_2)$

The column efficiency N is increased by the reduced size of the stationary phase particles. A column packed with small particles reaches its Van Deemter minimum at a higher flow rate than the one packed with the small particles the diffusion paths for the sample are short and reduce the broad broadening and hence increasing efficiency. The column efficiency can also be increased by increasing the length of the column. However, note because of the square root term in the above equation, doubling the length of the column will increase N by only 1.4 and not by a factor of 2.

The following example of the Resolution of R1 and R2 is shown in fig no.2.12.

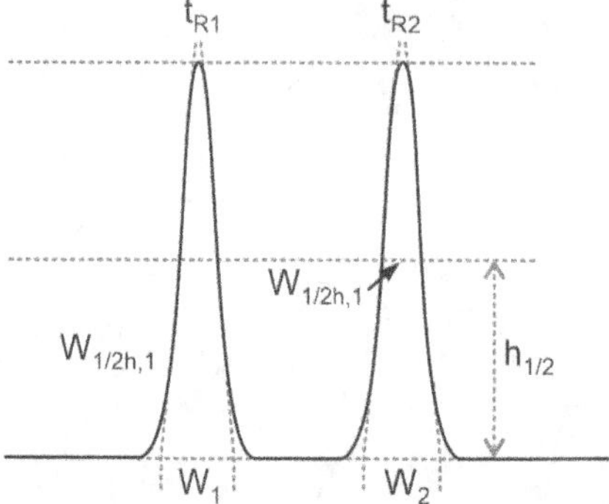

Fig. 2.12 Resolution of two peaks, R1 and R2.

The equation of Resolution is as follows

$$R_s = \frac{t_{R2} - t_{R1}}{1/2(W_1 + W_2)}$$

$$= 1.18 \times \frac{t_{R2} - t_{R1}}{W_{1/2h,1} + W_{1/2h,2}}$$

These are important terms used in representing peak information as follows,

1. Peak Base: An interpolation of the baseline between the Extremities of the peak.

2. Peak Area: The area enclosed by the peak and the peak base.

3. Peak Height: The distance from the peak maximum to the peak base.

4. Peak Width (tW): The magnitude of the peak base intercepted by the tangents to the inflection points of the peak.

5. Retention time (tR): The time between sample injection and the appearance of a solute peak at the detector of a chromatographic column.

6. Deadtime (tm): The time it takes for an unretained species (mobile phase) to pass through a column.

7. Adjusted Retention Time (tR) is the time solute spent in the stationary phase and equals to [tR- tm].

8. The Capacity Factor (k') is used to describe the migration rates of solutes on columns. It is defined as:

   For solute V1, kV1' = (tR,V1 – v0)/t0 ; = t'R,V1/v0

9. The Selectivity Factor (a) of a column for the two solutes V1 and V2 in a mixture is defined as a = k'V2/k'V1

The capacity factors K', as stated earlier, are related to the distributions of the sample in the mobile phase and stationary phases. K' is directly proportional to the volume occupied by the stationary phase, which in turn is related to the surface area (meter2gram-1) (m2g-1) of the particles. For similar conditions, a column packed with completely porous particles gives a larger K' than a column packed with porous-layer beads.

For solute V1,

$$kV1' = (tR,V1 - v0)/t0 \; ; \; = t'R,V1/v0$$

Also, particles with narrow pores produce a larger K' value than the wide pore material. These are some of the physical factors which may affect r', however, as pointed out earlier, for two components in a mixture to resolve, their K' must be different.

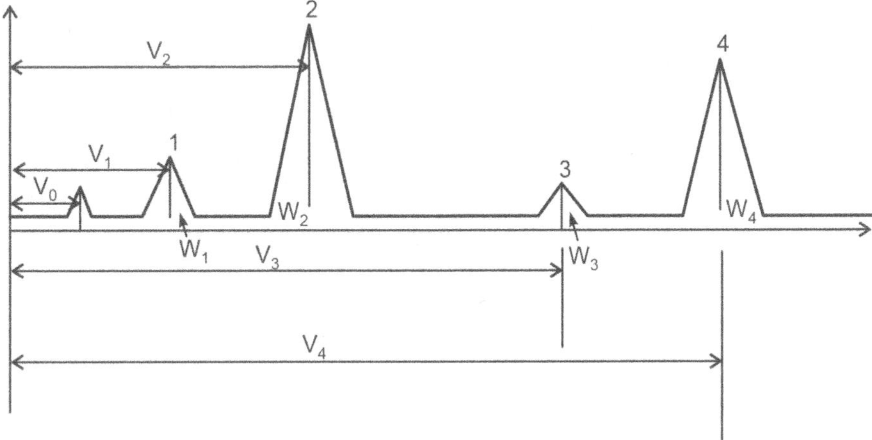

Fig. 2.13 Resolution of two peaks, R1 and R2.

The relative retention gives the assessment of this difference or the selectivity α, given by a = k'V2/k'V1. In practice, k' is calculated from the retention time as shown in No. fig. 2.13.

The most effective but also difficult way of improving resolution is to increase the selectivity α. The selectivity and, therefore, K' depends on the interaction of the sample molecules with the mobile and/or stationary phases. The type of interaction forces involved are depression forces, dipole-dipole interaction, hydrogen bonding, and π- π interactions. The ability of the sample molecule to interact with all four of these forces is referred to as the polarity of the sample. The solvent strength is directly related to its polarity such that solvent strength increases with increasing polarity. However, this generalisation for solvent is true for normal-phase or absorption chromatography. For reversed-phase chromatography, where the stationary phase is nonpolar, the solvent strength decreases with increasing polarity. The solvent is also regarded as strong if it eluates the sample with a shorter R' and weak if it increases its R'. Generally, chromatographic conditions are optimised to achieve for a two components mixture an optimum range of R' of between 2-5 and for a multi-component mixture R' of less than 10.

According to IP (1996), the capacity factor k' is calculated as follows

$$K' = V_1 - V_o / V_o$$

Where Vo = the distance along the baseline between the point of injection and the perpendicular dropped from the maximum of the peak of an unretained component.

V1 = the distance along the baseline between the point of injection and the perpendicular dropped from the maximum of the peak of interest.

$$Rs = 1.18 \, (V_2 - V_1) / \, W_1 + W_2$$

Where V_2 & V_1 = the distance along the baseline between the point of injection and the perpendicular dropped from the maximum of two adjacent peaks

W_1 & W_2 = the respective peak widths measured at half peak height.

$$Rs = \sqrt{N}/4 \qquad \times \qquad [\alpha-1]/\,\alpha \qquad \times \qquad [k'V2/(k'V2+1)]$$

Column efficiency	Selectivity	Capacity

THREE

MODES OF LIQUID CHROMATOGRAPHY (LC)

The selection of liquid chromatography (LC) mode for analysis or isolation of a given sample will essentially depend on its change, solubility and size. A vast majority of synthetic pharmaceuticals are water-soluble and have a molecular weight of less than 2000 daltons. The Indian Pharmacopoeia (1996) show the majority of HPLC methods for drug analysis are carried out using reversed-phase (RP) HPLC. For separation of synthetic and natural drug products, the methods of choice will be either normal phase (adsorption) chromatography, reversed-phase chromatography, and for very polar compounds, ion-exchange chromatography. However, for genetically engineered macromolecular pharmaceuticals and biotechnology products such as monoclonal antibodies, interferon, and tissue plasminogen activator, which are increasingly used in human medicine, the chromatographic separation of these products may require different LC modes from those used for synthetic drugs. The following decision trees illustrate the LC modes used for low molecular (<2000) weight drugs and high molecular weight (>20000) macromolecular drugs. The main subject of the book is the HPLC separation of small size pharmaceuticals and drug substances, and therefore, chromatographic separations of large molecules are described very briefly.

LC modes used in the production scale of isolation and purification of genetically engineered proteins from fermentation media may involve the following in downstream processing.

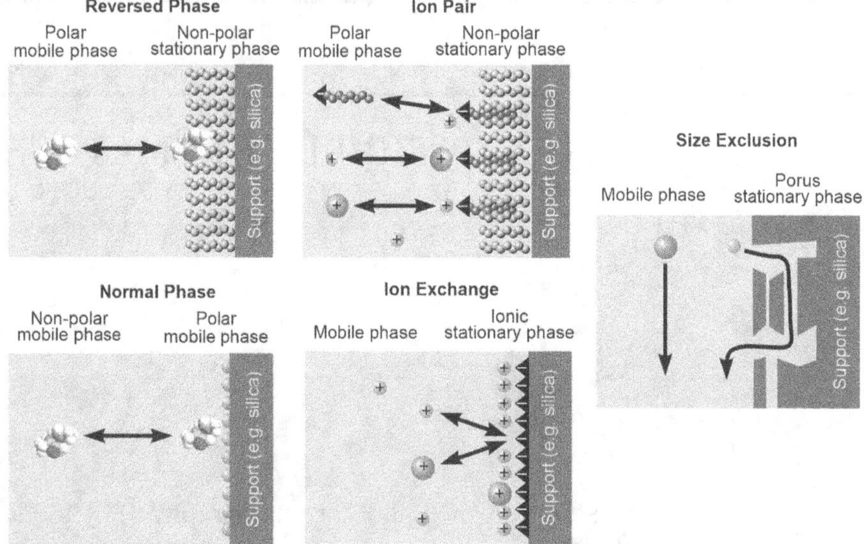

Fig. 3.1 Different Stationary Phases.

In the characterisation and quality control of purified protein, the following analytical scale LC modes may be involved.

This section briefly describes ion exchange, SEC, affinity, hydrophobic chromatography, and adsorption chromatography. As mentioned earlier, these LC modes are not frequently used for small synthetic pharmaceutical drugs.

A. Size exclusive chromatography (SEC)

The SEC technique is often referred to as gel permeation chromatography (GPC) if used with organic solvents and SEC if used with aqueous solvents. SEC is extensively used in the isolation and characterisation of high molecular weight proteins and peptides. The technique is simple and different from all other LC modes in that the separation is based on molecular size rather than on interaction mechanisms.

The stationary phases used in exclusion chromatography are porous particles of a closely controlled pore size. The sample molecules that are too large to diffuse into the pores are excluded, that is, they can travel only through the relatively wide channels between the stationary phase particles. The excluded molecules, therefore, emerge out of the column first. However, if molecules are small enough to penetrate all the available pores, then the whole of the mobile phase volume becomes available to them. These molecules are totally permeated and elute out of the column at last. Medium-sized molecules only use the part of the available pore volume, and they elute between the totally excluded and totally permeated molecules. The total volume of the mobile phase in the SEC column is the sum of the void volume (Vo), the volume outside the stationary phase particles and the volume within the pores of the particles or the interstitial volume (Vi). The totally excluded molecules must have a retention volume, Vo, and totally permeated have a retention volume of (Vo+Vi). Molecules of intermediate size will have a retention volume between Vo and (Vo+Vi). For estimating the molecular mass of proteins, the size exclusion column is first calibrated with proteins of known molecular mass (molecular weight markers). When the relative molecular mass of the marker, M, is plotted on a log scale against its retention volume, a calibration graph shown in Figure 3.5 is obtained.

SEC is based on the different interactions of solutes with the flowing mobile phase and the stagnant mobile phase.

- no true stationary phase is present in this system

- stagnant mobile phase acts as the "stationary phase."

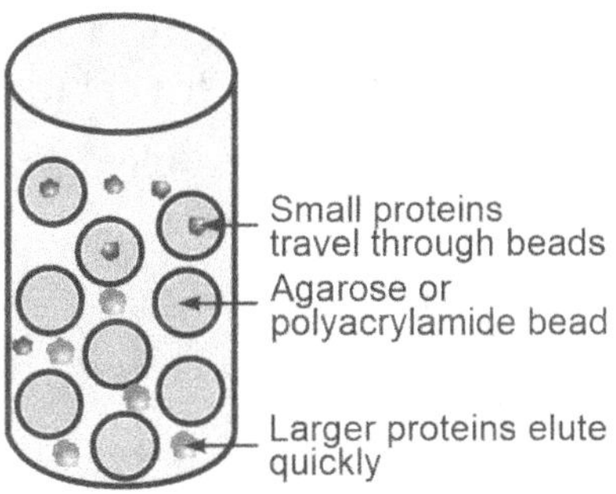

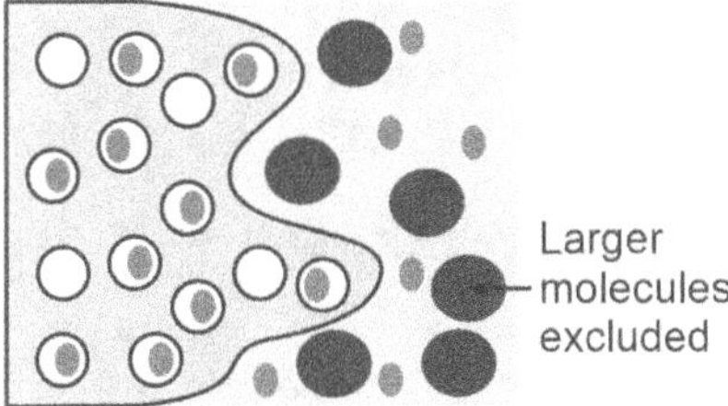

Molecular Exclusion Chromatography   **Fig. 3.2** Different Stationary Phases.

SEC is based on the use of a support material that has a certain range of pore sizes

- as solute travels through the support, small molecules can enter the pores while large molecules can not

- since the larger molecules sample a smaller volume of the column, they elute before the smaller molecules.
- separation based on size or molecular weight

From the elution volume of an unknown protein, its molecular weight is extrapolated from the calibration graph.

Since proteins may readily denature in organic solvents, the mobile phase for SEC separation of proteins is almost always aqueous or aqueous buffers.

B. Affinity Chromatography

Affinity chromatography exploits a unique biological specificity of the interaction between two compounds, such as antibodies and antigens. The technique is a major method of protein purification based on an interaction between biologically active materials, one of which is usually covalently coupled to an inert support. Some of the applications of affinity chromatography have been in the purification of antibodies, enzymes, hormones, receptors and viruses. Affinity chromatography may be used for either partial or final purification or separation of the desired sample from a large number of contaminating molecules in, for example, fermentation media.

Separates based on the use of immobilised biological molecules (and related compounds) as the stationary phase

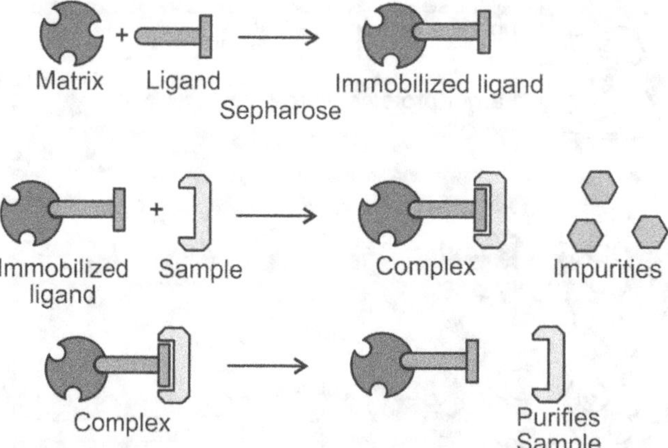

Fig. 3.3 Affinity Chromatography.

Based on the selective, reversible interactions that characterise most biological systems

- binding of an enzyme with its substrate or a hormone with its receptor

- immobilise one of a pair of interacting molecules onto a solid support
- Immobilised molecule on the column is referred to as the affinity ligand.

Two Main Types of Affinity Ligands Used in AC:

Table 3.1 High-specificity ligands compounds that bind to only one or a few very closely related molecules

Affinity Ligand	Retained Compounds
Antibodies	Antigens
Antigens	Antibodies
Inhibitors/Substrates	Enzymes
Nucleic Acids	Complimentary Nucleic acids

Table 3.2 General or group-specific ligands – molecules which bind to a family or class of related molecules

Affinity Ligand	Retained Compounds
Lectins	Glycoproteins, carbohydrates, membrane proteins
Triazine dyes	NADH- or NADPH Dependent Enzymes
Phenylboronic acid	*Cis*-Diol Containing Compounds
Protein A/Protein G	Antibodies
Metal Chelates	Metal-Binding Proteins & Peptides

Note: the affinity ligand does not necessarily have to be of biological origin

C. Ion Exchange Chromatography

Ion exchange chromatography is used for compounds with ionic or ionisable functional groups such as amino acids. With the introduction of ion-pair reversed-phase chromatography, the use of ion-exchange chromatography for small molecular weight pharmaceuticals has diminished considerably. The method is extensively used to separate proteins, peptides for sugar residues of glycoproteins and amino acids analysers (AA) use ion exchange columns to separate amino acids. Fully automated AA are still extensively used for examining the amino acid composition of proteins and peptides.

The principle of ion-exchange chromatography is similar to that of absorption chromatography in that the adsorbent in both methods bear active sites with which molecules interact for adsorption. In the case of adsorption or normal phase chromatography with silica as the adsorbent, silanol (Si-OH) is the active site. In the case of ion-exchange chromatography, the active sites are either positively charged (anion exchanger) or negatively charged (cation exchanger) groups.

Tables 3.3 and 3.4 lists some of the functional groups which are chemically bonded to a matrix, such as silica gel, polysaccharides, salt dextran gels or cross-linked polystyrene- divinyl benzene polymer.

Table 3.3 Cation exchanger

Functional groups	Formula
Carboxymethyl (CM)	$-OCH_2COO^-$
Sulphapropyl (SP)	$-OCH_2CH_2CH_2SO_2^-$
Methyl Sulphonate (S)	$-CH_2SO_2^-$

Table 3.4 Anion exchanger

Functional groups	Formula
Dimethyl Aminoethyl (DEAE)	$-OCH_2CH_2NH(C_2H_5)_2$
Quaternary amino ethyl (QAE)	$-OCH_2CH_2NHC_2H_5$
Quaternary Ammonium (Q)	$-OCH_2N(CH_3)_3$

- Reversible exchange of ionic species between the stationary phase and mobile phase
- Ionic species chemically bound to insoluble matrix serves as exchange site (adsorption)
- Insoluble matrix (M+) and counter ion (E-) as stationary phase
- Analyte ion (A-) in mobile phase

$$M+E- + A- \qquad M+A- + E-$$

- Silica based materials
  - Pellicular particles
- Organic materials
  - porous beads
  - styrene/divinylbenzene crosslinked co-polymers
  - methacrylic acid/divinylbenzene crosslinked co-polymers
- Inorganic materials

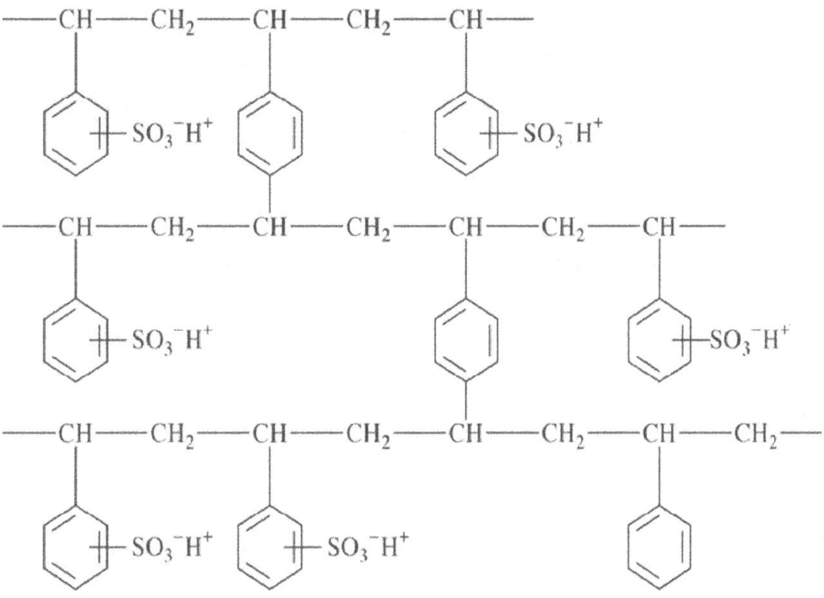

Fig. 3.4 Structure of polymer-based cation and anion exchanger.

IEC Stationary Phases

- Functional group addition through surface reactions with appropriate reagents to produce the desired cation or anion exchange resin
- Cation exchangers (strong & weak)
  - Acid functional groups
- Anion exchangers (strong & weak)
  - Basic functional groups

Resin Cross-linkage

- Pore size a degree of crosslinkage
- High degrees of Crosslinkage:
  - increase mechanical strength of the resin
  - decrease the degree of swelling
  - decrease the permeability of the resin

IEC Mobile Phases

- Aqueous solutions of salt or salts with a small % of organic modifier and perhaps a buffer

Retention & Selectivity Factors

- Size and shape of the solvated molecule

- Mobile phase pH
- Concentration & type of competing ion
- Addition of organic solvent to the mobile phase
- Column temperature

Cation M-A+ Bond Strengths

- Ce3+ > Al3+ >> Ba2+ > Pb2+ > Ca2+ > Ni2+ > Cu2+ > Mg2+ > UO22+ >> Tl+ > Ag+ > K+ > NH4+ > H+

Anion M+A- Bond Strengths

- Citrate > SCN- > CrO42- > SO42- > NO3- > Br- > CN- > Cl- > HCO3- > HCOO- > OH-

  Anion selectivities are not as rigidly defined as those of cations

Prediction of MxAy Bond Strengths

- Factors:
  - charge on the solute ion
  - size of the solvated ion
  - degree of resin crosslinkage
  - polarizability of the solute molecule
  - ion-exchange capacity of the resin
  - functional group on the resin
  - degree of interaction between the solute and the resin.

Ion Chromatography

- Separation of inorganic cations and anions and low molecular weight water-soluble organic acids and bases
- Non-suppressed IC methods
- Suppressed IC methods

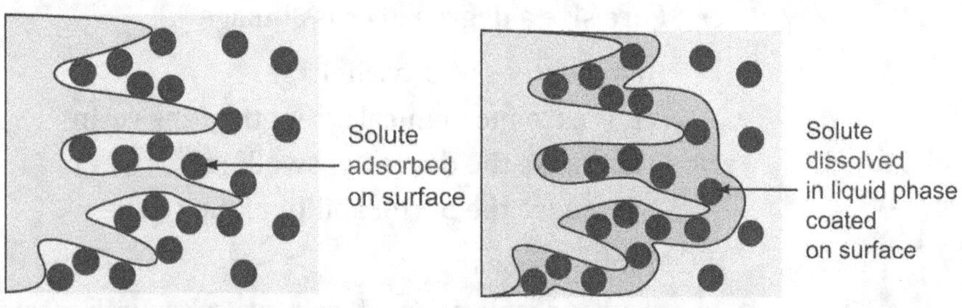

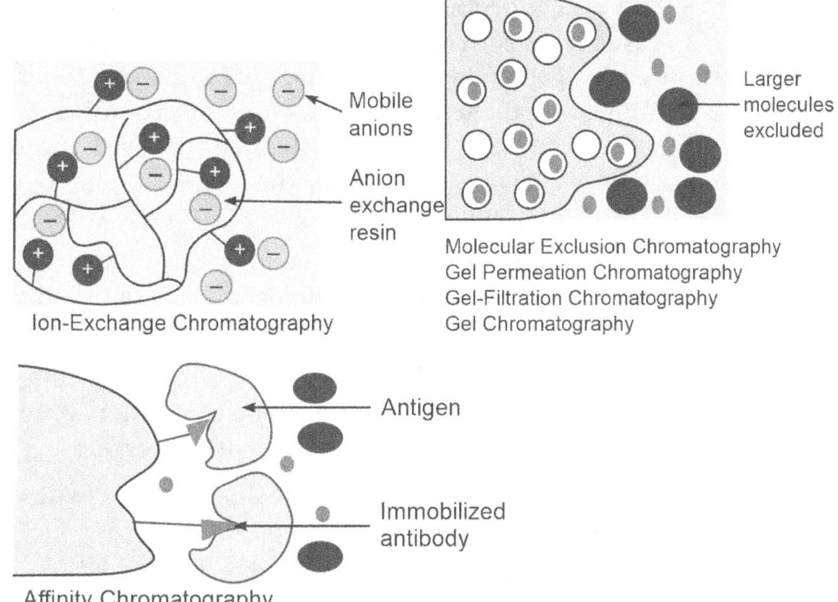

Fig. 3.5 Ion Exchange gel & Affinity Chromatography of Proteins.

D. Ion Exchange Chromatography of Proteins

Proteins and peptides are polymers composed of amino acid monomers whose amino groups (-NH2) and carboxyl (-COOH) groups have reacted to form an amide bond (-CONH).

The common amino acids may be separated into four groups:

Acidic   :   Cya (cysteic acid), Asp (Aspartic acid), The (Threonine), Ser (serine), Gly (glutamic acid)

Neutral :   Gly (glycine), Ala (alanine), Val(valine), Met (Methionine), Leu(Leucine), Ile(isoleucine)

Aromatic :   Phe (phenylalanine), Trp(tryptophan), try (tyrosine)

Basic   :   Lys (lysine), His (histidine), arg (arginine)

The overall acid-base properties of proteins depend on the ratio of acidic to basic amino acids in the molecules. Acidic proteins have an excess of acidic groups over basic groups and vice versa for basic proteins.

The ion exchange condition for separating a protein will depend on its isoelectric point (pI), the pH at which it carries no net charge. Depending upon the amino acid composition, a protein can be acidic (pI<6) or basic (pI>8). The choice of cation or anion exchanger, therefore, will depend on the pI of the protein under examination. At pH > pI, a protein is generally negatively charged and at pH<pI, it is usually positively charged. In theory, both anion and cation exchangers may be used for ion exchange separation of proteins. However, in general, acidic proteins (pI<6) are chromatographed when they are negatively charged and basic proteins (pI>8) when they are positively charged. The protein of pI between 6 and 8 can be chromatographed as either positive or negative species.

Chromatographic conditions for both anion and cation exchange separation of protein are almost always salt gradients of low to high salt concentrations. Aqueous conditions are always used to minimise the denaturation and hence the loss of potencies of proteins.

The charged groups that make up the stationary phase can be placed on several different types of support materials:

Cross-linked polystyrene resins: for use with the separation of inorganic ions and small organic ions

Carbohydrate-based resins: for low-performance separations of biological molecules (dextran, agarose, cellulose)

Silica-based supports: for high-performance separations of biological molecules

A strong mobile phase in IEC: contains a high concentration of a competing ion for the displacement of the sample ion from the stationary phase.

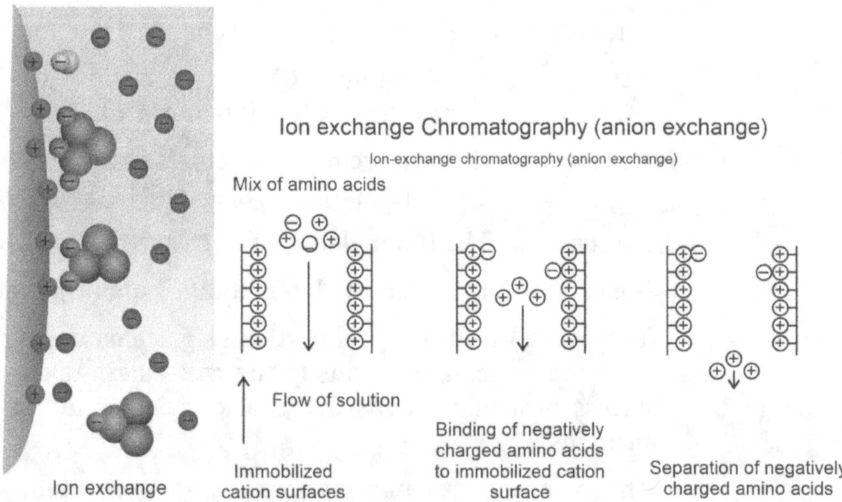

Fig. 3.6 Ion Exchange Chromatography.

cation exchange resin (Kex):

$Tl^+ > Ag^+ > Cs^+ > Rb^+ > K^+ > NH_4^+ > Na^+ > H^+ > Li^+$

$Ba^{2+} > Pb^{2+} > Sr^{2+} > Ca^{2+} > Ni^{2+} > Cd^{2+} > Cu^{2+} > Co^{2+} > Zn^{2+} > Mg^{2+} > UO_2^{2+}$

anion exchange resin (Kex):

$SO_4^{2-} > C_2O_4^{2-} > I^- > NO_3^- > Br^- > Cl^- > HCO_2^- > CH_3CO_2^- > OH^- > F^-$

or

- a solvent that has a pH which decreases ionization of the analyte or stationary phase

HYDROPHOBIC INTERACTION CHROMATOGRAPHY (HIC)

Hydrophobic Interaction Chromatography (HIC) is sometimes used to separate the enzymes and proteins where maintenance of biological activity is essential. HIC has a hydrophilic matrix which is lightly substituted by propyl, butyl or phenyl groups.

In HIC, the proteins are induced to bind weakly with the hydrophobic stationary phase using a high ionic strength mobile phase. Adsorbed proteins are then selectively desorbed during a linear descending gradient, finishing with a very low ionic buffer or water. The gradient conditions used for HIC are opposite to those used for ion-exchange chromatography of proteins.

NORMAL PHASE CHROMATOGRAPHY (NPC)

The chromatographic mode is referred to as normal, where the stationary phase is more polar than the mobile phase. In case of silica, for example, the adsorption sites on the surface of the silica are highly polar silinol (-SiOH) groups. The strength of interaction between the silinol group and solute molecule gets stronger with the increasing polarity of the solute. Therefore to increase the retention (R') of the sample, one would need to use a weak (low polarity) solvent and to decrease the retention (R') would require a (polar) solvent. In case of silica, a hydrocarbon such as hexane is a weak solvent, and water is a strong solvent, in fact, water is so strong a solvent that a small amount of it in the mobile phase would readily displace solute from the silica surface. The water contents of the mobile phase in adsorption chromatography using silica gel have a more profound effect on chromatography than for any other modes of chromatography. One of the problems associated with the use of silica for chromatography is its limited pH stability. Above pH 8, silica becomes increasingly soluble, which shortens the lifetime of the HPLC column. It is therefore not advisable under normal circumstances to use any silica-based packing at pH values less than pH 2 or greater than 7. the surface areas of the silica particles used for HPLC are high of the order of $200\text{-}600m^2g^{-1}$.

The other materials used for Normal phase chromatography (NPC) are alumina and zirconium oxide, and titanium oxide to a minor extent. The polar, water-soluble solutes such as pharmaceutical drugs are strongly held on base silica. The method is more useful for solutes of low polarity. However, bonded phase and normal phase chromatography are often used to separate various compounds of medium polarity.

As shown in table no.4.1, Solvent strength in Normal phase chromatography (NPC).

The polarity and strength of pure solvents have been defined in various ways. One measure of polarity is the solubility parameter (δ) which was suggested by Hildebrand. This is defined as the square root of solvents vaporization energy (ΔE) divided by its molar volume (V).

Table 4.1 Solubility parameter (δ) and other physicochemical properties of solvents used in HPLC.

Solvent	δ	Refractive Index	UV (nm) cut off	Boiling Point
Hexane	14.9	1.378	210	69.0
Diethylether	15.5	1.353	220	34.6
Carbon tetra chloride	17.8	1.466	265	76.8
Tatrahydrofuran	19.1	1.407	280	64.7
Chloroform	19.1	1.443	245	61.3
Acetone	20.2	1.359	330	56.2
Acetonitrile	23.9	1.344	210	81.6
Methanol	29.4	1.329	210	64.6
water	47.8	1.333	200	100.0

$$\delta = \Delta E/E$$

Based on their δ values, table no.4.2. rank solvents are most often used in Normal phase chromatography. Water, as the most polar solvent, has the highest δ value. One of the difficulties with this type of solvent classification suggests that solvents with similar δ values would also be similar. The problem is shown by Chloroform (δ 19.1) which is water-immiscible, and acetone (δ 20.2) which is water-miscible. To overcome this discrepancy, Snyder proposed solvent polarity index P' and three other parameters- Xe (a proton acceptor parameter), Xd (a proton donor parameter) and Xn (a dipole parameter) to define solvent strengths. Table no.4.3. shows polarity parameters of some solvents used in HPLC based on the Snyder polarity indicator.

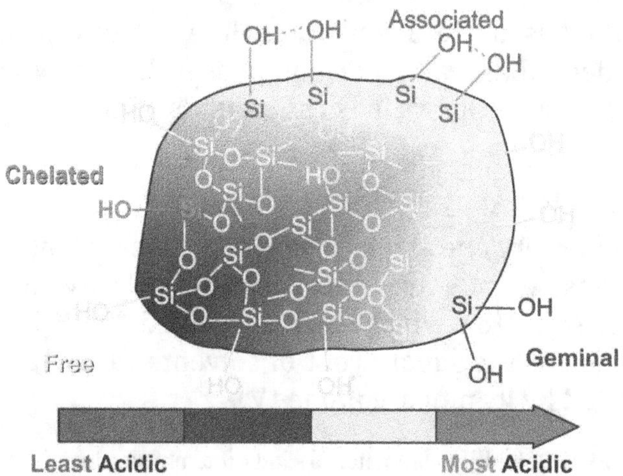

Fig. 4.1 Nature of Stationary Phase.

Table 4.2 Snyder polarity index for solvents used in HPLC.

Solvent	P'	Xe	Xd	Xn	Group
Hexane	0.1	-	-	-	-
Diethylether	2.8	0.53	0.13	0.34	I
Methanol	5.1	0.48	0.22	0.31	II
Ethanol	4.3	0.52	0.19	0.29	II
n-propanol	4	0.54	0.19	0.27	II
Isopropanol	3.4	0.56	0.18	0.25	II
Tatrahydrofuran	4	0.38	0.2	0.42	III
Acetic acid	6.2	0.39	0.31	0.3	IV
Dichloromethane	3.1	0.29	0.18	0.53	V
Acetonitrile	5.8	0.31	0.27	0.42	VI
Acetone	5.1	0.35	0.23	0.42	VI
Toluene	2.4	0.25	0.28	0.47	VII
Chloroform	4.1	0.25	0.41	0.33	VII
Water	10.2	0.37	0.37	0.25	VIII

The main advantage of the Snyder system is that it allows solvents to be grouped according to the type of interactions in which they take part. Solvents of the same chemical type have similar values for the selectivity parameters - Xe, Xd and Xn even though their P' values are different (e.g. four alcohols are listed above). Plotting the solvent selectivity parameters on the triangular diagram gives representation, as shown in fig. 4.2. All of the common solvents fall into one of eight groups represented as shown in Table no. 4.3.

Table 4.3 Members of groups I-VII

Group	Members
I	Aliphatic Ethers
II	Aliphatic alcohols
III	Pyridine derivatives, THF, sulphoxide
IV	Glycols, acetic acid
V	Dichloromethane
VI	Aliphatic esters. Ketones, nitriles, dioxane
VII	Aromatic hydrocarbons, halogenated aromatics, aromatic ethers, nitro compounds
VIII	water

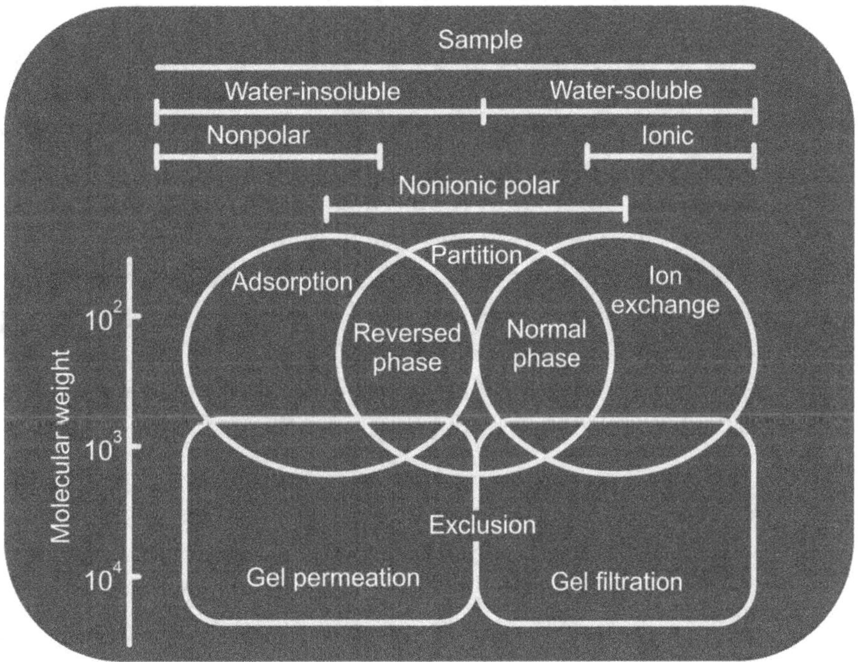

Fig. 4.2 Systemic diagram of Chromatographic Methods.

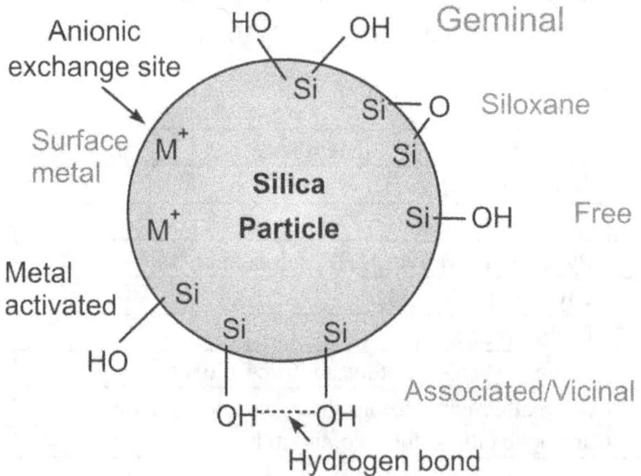

Fig. 4.3 Types of Silanol Groups.

As pointed out earlier, retention in NPC is based on the adsorption process, whereas retention in RPC is believed to resemble a partition process. This is illustrated in fig 4.8 for the retention of sample molecule S from a mobile phase containing polar solvent molecules M. the surface of the column packing is initially covered with a layer of solvent molecule M for retention of the sample molecules S to occur, it requires the displacement of molecules M to provide space for the adsorption of S. The polar species S and M thus gets adsorbed and described by active sites. The types of Silanol groups and their bonding is as shown in fig.no.4.3.

Compounds with very polar groups and polar solvents interact and adsorb strongly onto the active polar sites like silanol. Strongly adsorbed molecules are then referred to as localized. Localization of polar solvent molecules allows better selectivity control. Based on their experimental adsorption solvent strength parameter ε^0, yet another solvent strength scale for NPC has been derived. Table no.4.4. list ε^0 of commonly used solvents for NPC.

Table 4.4 NPC solvent strength ε^0 and selectivity.

Solvent	ε^0	Localization	Basic
Hexane	0	No	Solvent basicity is irrelevant for non-localizing solvents
Heptane	0	No	=
Chloroform	0.26	No	=
Methylene chloride	0.30	No	=
2 propyl ether	0.32	Minor	=
1,2 dichloro ethane	0.34	No	=
ethyl ether	0.38	Yes	Yes
Methyl t butyl ether	0.48	Yes	Yes
Ethyl acetate	0.48	Yes	No
Dioxane	0.51	Yes	Yes
Acetonitrile	0.52	Yes	No
Tetrahydro furan	0.53	Yes	Yes
1 or 2 propanol	0.60	Yes	Presence of proton donor group
Methanol	0.70	Yes	=

MOBILE PHASE SELECTIVITY

In NPC, a weak (non-polar) solvent A and a strong (polar) solvent B are first selected and then blended to obtain a mobile phase composition to maximize resolution. Mobile phase selectivity can also be offered by varying per cent B or changing to a strong solvent.

Regardless of the mobile phase or stationary phase used, sample retention in NPC increases as the polarity of the mobile phase decrease. The stationary phase may be silica, alumina or phases bonded with cyano, diol or amino functional groups.

NPC USING BONDED PHASE

In addition to silica, chemically bonded silica with cyano, amino and diol groups, the so-called polar bonded phase (PBP), are also used for NPC. The reactions used for the synthesis of these PBP are shown in Fig.no. 4.4 and table no. 4.4. To reiterate, NPC is defined as the chromatography in which the stationary phase is more polar than the mobile phase. The mobile phase in the NPC is usually a mixture of organic solvents without added water. Sample retention increases as the polarity of the mobile phase decrease.

In case of silica, the adsorption sites are polar silanol groups. In PBP, cyano, amino and diol columns, the bonded phase ligands are the adsorption sites. The selectivity of silica, cyano, diol and amino column is quite different from each other. Basic compounds are preferentially retained on amino and diol columns compared to cyano columns, whereas dipolar compounds are more strongly retained on cyano columns compared to amino and diol columns. Silica has better selectivity for the separation of isomers; however, in case of silica, the control of the mobile phase is more critical than for the PBP phases

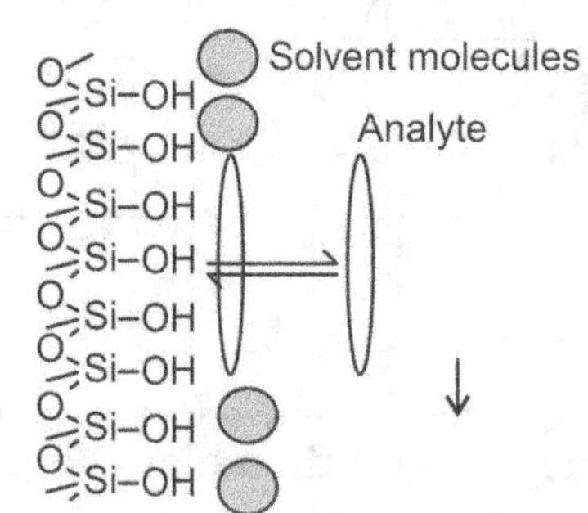

Fig. 4.4 Normal Phase Stationary Phase.

REVERSED-PHASE CHROMATOGRAPHY (RPC)

As the term suggests, in RPC, the nature of the phases is reversed from those used in the NPC. In **RPC,** the stationary phase is less polar than the mobile phase. This reversal is achieved by altering the polar nature of the silanol groups of silica into non-polar groups. Silica-based packing is still the most popular support used in **RPC.** The polar silanol groups are chemically modified to give non-polar hydrophobic hydrocarbonaceous support such as octadecyl silica (ODS). Fig.no. 5.1. show reactions with chlorosilanes used to prepare polymeric or monomeric stationary phases. By modifying the side chain (R) on the organosilane, a wide variety of bonded stationary phases have been produced commercially. Table no.5.1. list some of the phases which have been prepared by the chemical modification of the silanol groups of silica.

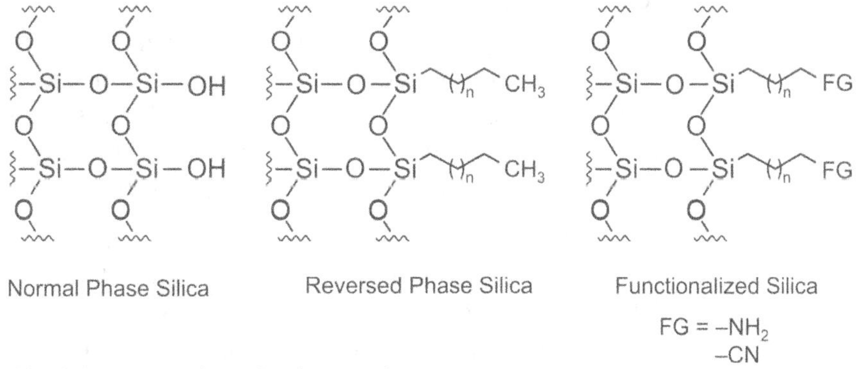

Fig. 5.1 Reverse Phase Stationary Phase.

Table 5.1 Functional groups in chemically modified silicas.

Group	Formula
Octadecyl	$(CH_2)_{17}CH_3$
Octyl	$(CH_2)_7CH_3$
Hexyl	$(CH_2)_5CH_3$
Butyl	$(CH_2)_3CH_3$
Phenyl	C_6H_5

Table 5.1 *Contd...*

Amino	NH_2
Amino propyl	$CH_2CH_2CH_2NH_2$
Nitro	NO_2
Nitrile	$--C\equiv N$

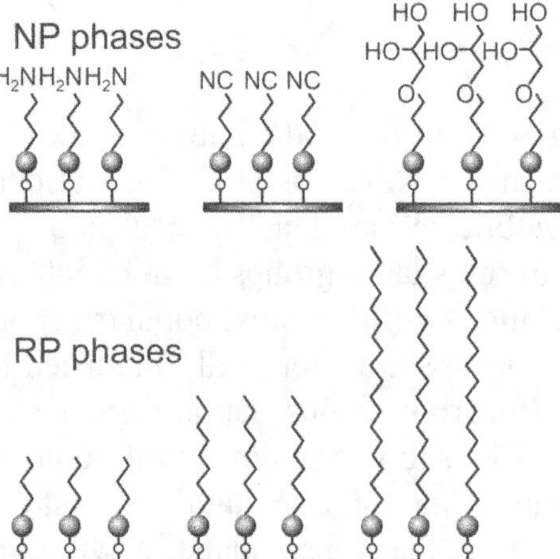

Fig. 5.2 Normal Phase & Reverse Phase Stationary Phase

In the reversed HPLC of polar drug substances, the mobile phase generally consists of a mixture of water or aqueous buffer solutions with various water-miscible solvents such as alcohols. Theoretically, the highest separation selectivity is achieved when the polarity difference between the mobile phase and the stationary phase is the greatest. In practice, the solvent strength of the mobile phase is adjusted with the hydrophobicity of the stationary phase for a given solute to elute with K' value between 2 to 10.

By virtue of the high polarity of water, RPC is suitable for analysing a much wider range of polarity of compounds than NPC. This wide range of solute polarity and compatibility with aqueous samples explains why RPC accounts for most of the present-day applications in the pharmaceutical industry. The most popular reversed-phase column used for drug substances is ODS ($R=C_{18}H_{37}$), followed by octyl ($R=C_8H_{17}$). Short alkyl chain phases such as butyl ($R=C_4H_9$) and propyl ($R=C_3H_7$) are used less frequently to analyse synthetic drug substances.

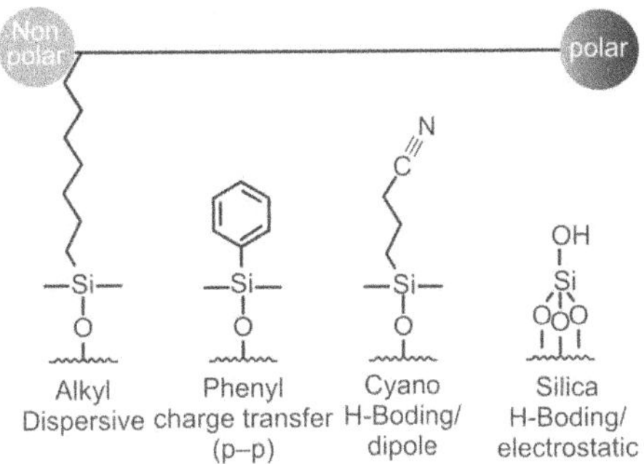

Fig. 5.3 Normal Phase & Reverse Phase Stationary Phase.

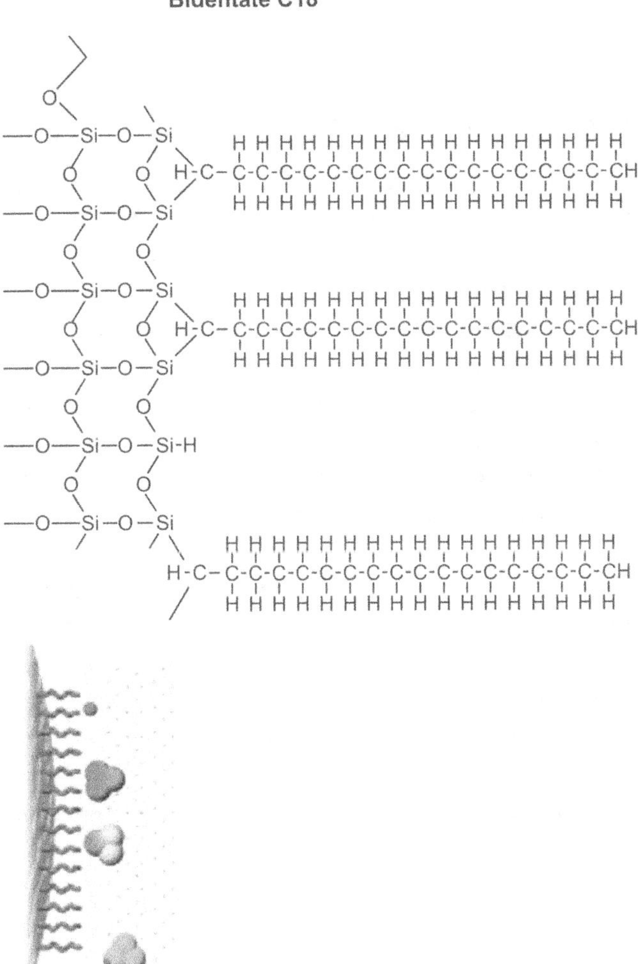

Fig. 5.4 Reverse Phase Stationary Phase C18 Column.

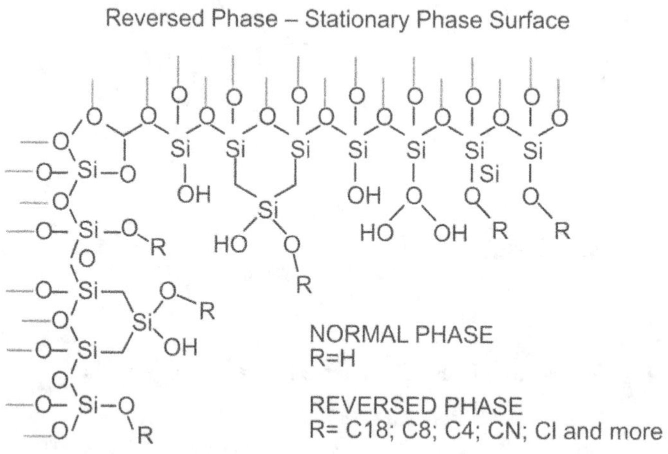

Reversed Phase – Stationary Phase Surface

Fig. 5.5 Normal Phase & Reverse Phase Stationary Phase.

A. Polymeric and Monomeric Bonded Phases and end-capping

The reaction schemes shown in fig 5.5 illustrate a one to one relationship between the silanol group and the derivatising reagent, resulting in one r group for each silanol. This type of phase is referred to as a monomeric. By using a trichloroalkylsilane rather than monochloroalkylsilane as the reagent, the product resulting from one to one reaction can further react with either a nearby silanol or another chloroalkylsilane leading to the build-up of several layers. This type of stationary phase is termed polymeric. Because of the steric hindrance, not all the silanols on the silica will react with the derivatising reagent, leaving unreacted residual silanols. Any residual silanol will impart polar character to the stationary phase, which will cause peak tailing of polar compounds, especially bases. To overcome this problem, the bonded phase material is further reacted with small trimethyl silane, which because of its smaller size, will have better access to unreacted silanols. This procedure is called end-capping. Many manufacturers claim to have either 100 % end-capped or fully end-capped packing materials. In reality, there will still be some unreacted silanol groups remaining.

Many of the problems associated with using ODS columns for the analysis of the compounds may be traced to the presence of residual silanol groups. The use of the acidic mobile phase reduces the effect of the silanol groups.

The pKa of silanol is approximately 3.5, so in acidic conditions, silanol will be protonated, thus reducing the ionisation. Another mobile phase modification is to add 30 to 50 mm of triethylamine for analysis of basic compounds, ammonium acetate for acidic compounds and trimethylamine acetate for unknown. The addition of 10 mm of dimethyloctyl amine or dimethyl octyl amine acetate may reduce the difference in the chromatographic properties of ODS columns for basic compounds.

B. Carbon load and retention

In the reversed-phase chromatography, hydrophobic interactions between the stationary phases, mobile phases and sample molecules dominate the retention. The retention of the alkyl bonded phases is greatly influenced by the carbon loading, generally expressed as the percentage. The carbon loading of the stationary phase depends on the relative surface coverage and the chain length of the bonded functional groups. It also depends on the surface area of the silica support and method of manufacture- monomeric, polymeric and end-capping. For an ODS bonded phase, the carbon loading may vary from approximately 10 to 20 %, for an octyl silane bonded phase, the value is more typically 5 to 10 %. As the chain length of the alkyl group (R) increases, the solute retention time will also increase. The higher the carbon load, the more hydrophobic will be the stationary phase.

C. Reversed-phase HPLC using polymeric support

Silica-based stationary phases are still most popular in the RP-HPLC of drug substances. However, adsorbents based on the polymer (styrene-divinylbenzene copolymer) are slowly gaining ground. The main disadvantage of the silica-based support is the pH stability of the silica gel. In alkaline pH, silica dissolves slowly, which could shorten the usability of the HPLC column significantly. The effective range of the mobile phase pH for silica-based HPLC column is 2 to 7. the polymer-based RP HPLC column is stable over a wide pH range, commonly quoted as from pH 1 to 13. This allows a much greater choice of mobile phases than would be advisable with a silica-based RP-HPLC column, especially for separating the basic compounds. The ionisation of bases becomes possible by operating at high pH values. The main drawbacks of polymeric supports are their reduced polymeric efficiencies and their low mechanical resistance to high pressure. The cross-linking process used to manufacture the polymeric phase (fig.no.5.1) produces rigid, spherical particles with well-controlled pore size. This makes them ideal for use in size exclusion chromatography as well.

D. Solvent strength and elutropic series for RPC

The polarities of the solvents discussed for the normal phase earlier are reversed for RPC. Water, for example, for RPC, is the weakest solvent. Retention in the RPC is controlled by the concentration of water in the mobile phase and decreases with an increase in the concentration of water. Retention in RPC is believed to resemble a partition process rather than the adsorption process for NPC. The solute-solvent interaction which arise from proton acceptor (Xe parameter), proton donor (Xd parameter) and dipole (Xn parameter) discussed in solvent table 4.4 provides the basis for mobile phase optimisation procedures in RPC systems. The elutropic series for commonly used solvents in RPC is shown in table no.5.2.

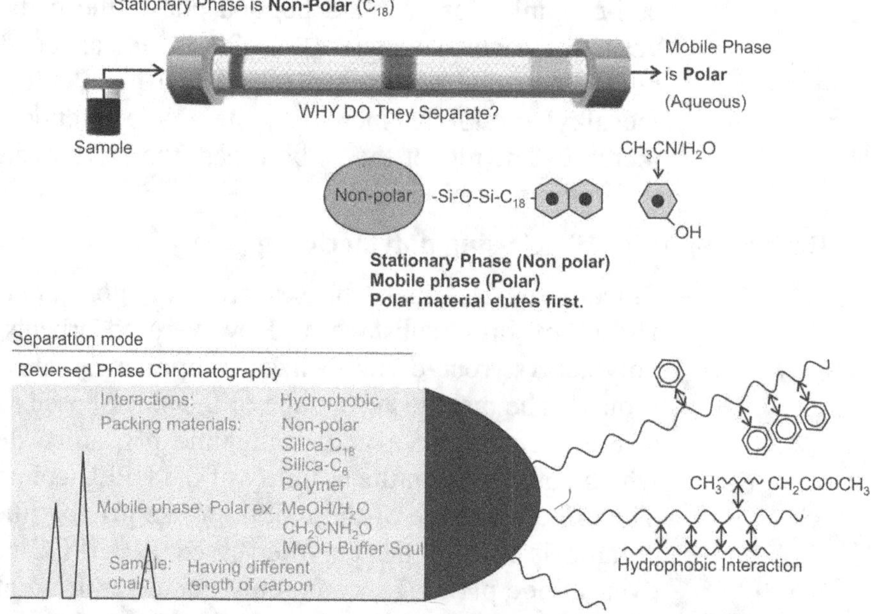

Fig. 5.6 Types of Stationary Phases.

Table 5.2 Elutropic Series For RP-HPLC

Water	Decreasing polarity
Methanol	
Acetonitrile	
Acetone	
Ethanol	Increasing elution power
2 propanol	
Dimethylformamide	
1 propanol	
Dioxane	
Tetrahydrofuran	

Table 5.3 Comparison of RPLC & NPLC

Type	*Stationary phase*	*Weak mobile phase*	*Stationary phase*
RPLC	Non-polar	Polar liquid	Non-polar
NPLC	polar	Non-polar liquid	polar

The requirement that the solvent is miscible with water significantly limits the number of organic modifiers suitable for RPC. The suitability of the solvents shown in table no. 5.2 is further reduced by the prohibitive cost of the ethanol, the high UV cut off of acetone, high viscosity, and UV cut off of dimethylformamide and the high viscosity of propanol. Dioxane has solvent strength similar to that of acetonitrile. Therefore, in practice, the organic modifiers commonly used for RPC are methanol, acetonitrile and tetrahydrofuran.

E. Ion pair reversed-phase HPLC

For inferior ionic compounds, ion-exchange chromatography was the only viable option, but now fairly polar compounds can be separated by ion-pair RP-HPLC. The columns used for RP-HPLC and ion pair chromatography are the same. However, from a practical point of view, it is advisable to dedicate a separate column for ion pair chromatography. In the separation of ionic compounds by ion-pair chromatography, two approaches have been described.

The first approach involves the adjustment of the pH of the mobile phase so that the compound under examination is in a neutral or unionised form. This is referred to as ionic suppression. In general, the retention of a neutral form of an ionisable compound will be greater than the ionised form. The effects of the nature of the mobile phase and the stationary phase on the retention of the ionic compounds are essentially the same as the neutral compounds. When using silica based columns, the ion suppression method is limited to the mobile phase pH range of 2 to 7.

The second approach to influence the retention of the ionic compounds on RP-HPLC involves ion-pair extraction techniques. In this technique, the pH of the mobile phase is generally adjusted so that the compound or compounds of interest are in their ionised form. The retention is then manipulated by the addition of an oppositely charged ion pairing agents to the mobile phase. Ion-pairing agents form a coulombic complex which behaves as an electrical neutral and non-polar compound, as shown below.

Sample + counter ion ------ [sample - counter ion]

Sample + counter ion ------ [sample - counter ion]

Ion pairing agents have a negligible effect on neutral species but affect all charged species in the sample mixture. The method can be used to separate ionic and nonionic compounds in the same sample. Some commonly used counter ions for acids and bases in RP-HPLC are

Acidic compounds: quaternary amines such as tetramethyl-ammonium hydroxide (TMAH), tetrabutylammonium hydroxide (TBAH), Tertiary amines, e.g. trictylamine.

Basic compounds: Perchloric acid, alkyl and aryl sulphonates such as methane, pentane, heptane and camphorsulphonic acid.

The mobile phase pH for all counter ions should be kept between 2 to 7 when using a silica-based reversed-phase column. The concentration of ion pair reagent is usually kept in the 50-200mm range. The retention of the compounds in the ion-pair reversed-phase HPLC is affected by the concentration of the ion pairing reagents and their size. E. g. switching from methane to heptane sulphonic acid as a counter ion while keeping all other conditions constant would result in the increase of the retention time of the compound under examination. The retention time should also be adjusted by changing the amount of organic solvent in the mobile phase.

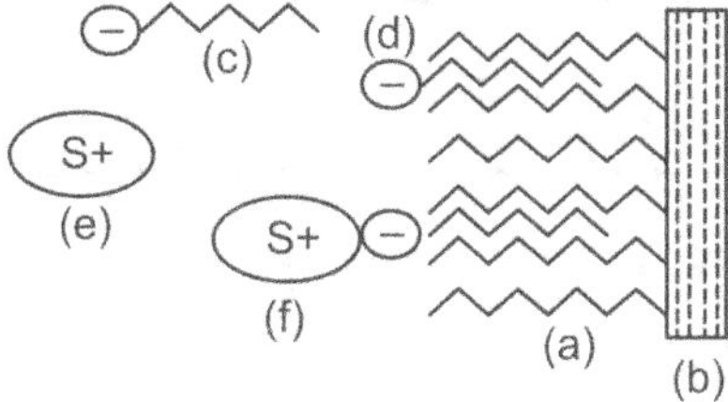

Fig. 5.7 Types of Stationary Phases.

TYPES OF STATIONARY PHASES

(a) Bonded Phase

(b) Stationary Phase

(c) Ion-pair reagent in mobile Phase

(d) Ion-pair reagent adsorbed to Stationary Phase

(e) Sample ion free in mobile Phase

(f) Sample retained on the column by ion-pair mechanism.

In reversed-phase chromatography, ionic compounds are usually not retained by the hydrophobic stationary phase.

- By adding an ion-pair reagent with an ionic end and a hydrophobic tail to the mobile Phase, the hydrophobic tail of the reagent gets retained by the stationary phase. Thus an ion-exchange group forms on the surface of the stationary phase.

The samples ion exchanges with the counter ion of the ion-pair reagent retained by the stationary phase, thus resulting in greater retention of the sample.

RETENTION MECHANISM

- **Two possible retention process**
  1. **Partition model**
  2. **Adsorption model**

Partition Model: In this model, the ion-pairing agent is present in the mobile phase. The analyte interacts with the ion-pairing agent in the mobile phase first. It forms the ion pair, which is relatively non-polar and partitioned into the stationary Phase and gets retained.

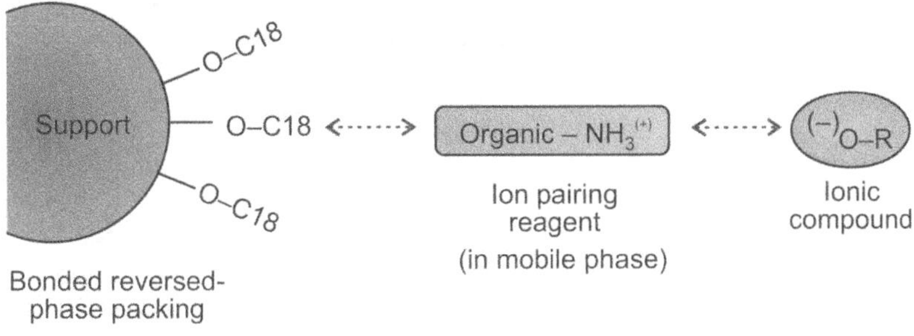

Fig. 6.1 Partition type of ion-pairing Stationary Phases.

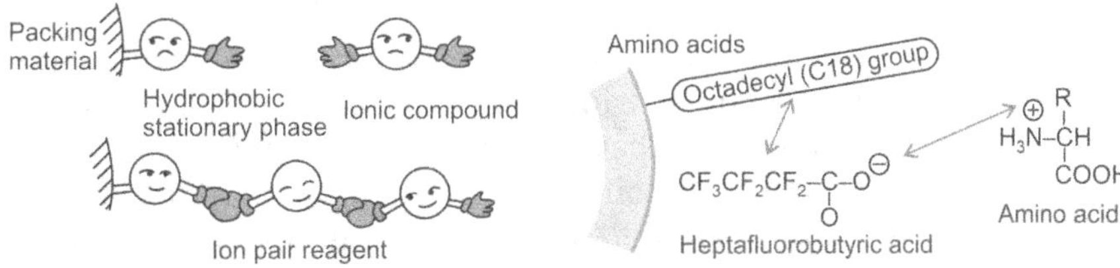

Fig. 6.2 Adsorption types of ion-pairing stationary phases.

ADSORPTION MODEL

The ion-pairing agent present in the mobile Phase gets adsorbed into the non-polar stationary Phase due to its lipophilic alkyl chain. As a result, the ion-pairing reagent forms a pseudo-ion-exchange layer on the surface of the stationary phase. The analyte interacts with the ion-pairing agent presented on the surface to form an ion-pair and gets retained.

A (mobile phase) + R⁺X (stationary Phase) ⇌ A R⁺(stationary Phase) + X⁻

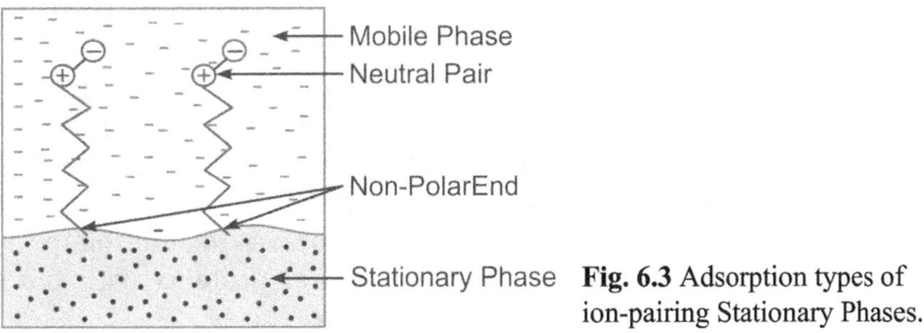

Fig. 6.3 Adsorption types of ion-pairing Stationary Phases.

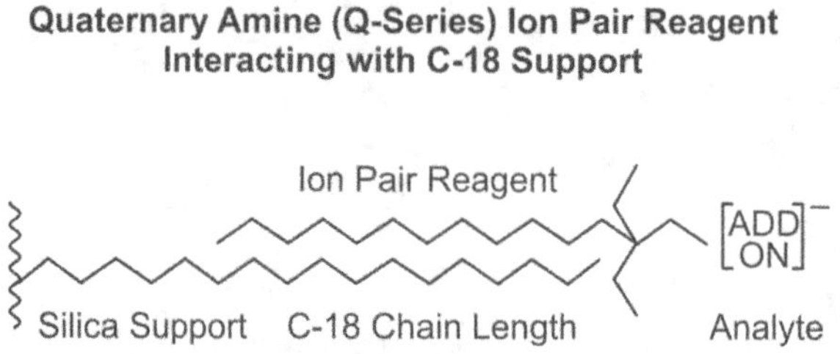

**Quaternary Amine (Q-Series) Ion Pair Reagent
Interacting with C-18 Support**

Ion Pair Reagent

Silica Support   C-18 Chain Length   Analyte

Fig. 6.4 Quaternary amine type of ion-pairing reagents.

REVERSED-PHASE CHROMATOGRAPHY OF PROTEINS AND PEPTIDES

The use of reversed-phase HPLC for protein and peptides separations has become widespread recently. Most literature report shows optimisation have been approached by two routes- mobile phase manipulation on a given stationary phase or selection of a reversed-phase packing. Most separations are carried out by using low pH mobile phases (pH about 2) that contain 0.1% trifluoroacetic acid (TFA), 0.1 M phosphate or acetate buffers as the aqueous Phase and acetonitrile or propan-1-ol as the organic phase. Almost all separations require gradient elution. The use of TFA as an ion-pairing agent has been popular because of its volatility and effectiveness as a solubilising agent for proteins. Other perfluoro carboxylic acids have also been found to have desirable selectivity.

In addition to the mobile Phase and the alkyl ligand, the pore size of the silica matrix of reversed-phase packing plays a significant role in separating the proteins. Silica-based reversed-phase support used for proteins are wide pore (pore size 20-30nm) and short bonded alkyl chain (propyl and butyl). For the separation of small peptide fragments resulting from proteolytic digests, narrow pore (6-10nm) size silica with a long alkyl chain (octyl and octadecyl) may be used.

Since the separation of proteins and peptides by RP-HPLC invariably involves gradients of aqueous/organic phases, the organic phases used in the mobile phases may denature the proteins and therefore destroy their biological potencies. Therefore, the method is generally used for the analytical separation of proteins rather than for the preparative purification of proteins. In addition to the organic solvent denaturation, the interaction of proteins with the stationary Phase may destroy their biological potencies

REVERSE PHASE LIQUID CHROMATOGRAPHY (RPLC)

Partition chromatography, where the stationary phase is the non-polar reverse polarity of normal Phase LC retains non-polar compounds most strongly, a weak mobile phase is a polar liquid: water and a strong mobile phase is more non-polar liquid: methanol or acetonitrile

The stationary phase must have low miscibility with the mobile phase, so the stationary phase is not dissolved from the column examples of liquid RPLC stationary phases:

< heptane < squalene < hydrocarbon polymers < dimethyl-polysiloxane

HIGH-PERFORMANCE LIQUID CHROMATOGRAPHY (HPLC)

Chromatography is a technique to separate mixtures of substances into their components based on their molecular structure and molecular composition. This involves a stationary phase (a solid or a liquid supported on a solid) and a mobile phase (a liquid or a gas). The mobile phase flows through the stationary phase and carries the components of the mixture with it. Sample components that display stronger interactions with the stationary phase will move more slowly through the column than components with weaker interactions. This difference in rates causes the separation of various components. Chromatographic separations can be carried out using a variety of stationary phases, including immobilized silica on glass plates (thin-layer chromatography), volatile gases (gas chromatography), paper (paper chromatography) and liquids (liquid chromatography).

INTRODUCTION OF HIGH-PERFORMANCE LIQUID CHROMATOGRAPHY

High-performance liquid chromatography (HPLC) is basically a highly improved form of column liquid chromatography. Instead of a solvent being allowed to drip through a column under gravity, it is forced through under high pressures of up to 400 atmospheres. That makes it much faster. All chromatographic separations, including HPLC, operate under the same basic principle; separation of a sample into its constituent parts because of the difference in the relative affinities of different molecules for the mobile phase and the stationary phase used in the separation. High Price Liquid Chromatography due to high-cost factors.

A. Types of HPLC

There are the following variants of HPLC, depending upon the phase system (stationary) in the process:

1. **Normal Phase HPLC**: This method separates analytes based on polarity. NP-HPLC uses a polar stationary phase and a non-polar mobile phase. Therefore, the stationary phase is usually silica. Typical mobile phases are hexane, methylene chloride, chloroform, diethyl ether, and mixtures. Polar samples are thus retained on the polar surface of the column, packing longer than less polar materials.

2. **Reverse Phase HPLC:** The stationary phase is non-polar (hydrophobic) in nature, while the mobile phase is a polar liquid, such as mixtures of water and methanol or acetonitrile. It works on the principle of hydrophobic interactions; hence the more non-polar the material is, the longer it will be retained.

3. **Size-exclusion HPLC:** The column is filled with a material with precisely controlled pore sizes, and the particles are separated according to their molecular size. Larger molecules are rapidly washed through the column; smaller molecules penetrate inside the porous of the packing particles and elute later.

4. **Ion-Exchange HPLC:** The stationary phase has an ionically charged surface of opposite charge to the sample ions. This technique is used almost exclusively with ionic or ionizable samples. The stronger the charge on the sample, the stronger it will be attracted to the ionic surface and, thus, the longer it will take to elute. The mobile phase is an aqueous buffer, where both pH and ionic strength are used to control elution time.

B. Types of Elution Methods in HPLC

Elution of solute is carried out by two methods in HPLC as follows.

1. **Isocratic elution:** A separation that employs a single solvent or solvent mixture of constant composition.

2. **Gradient elution:** Here, two or more solvent systems that differ significantly in polarity are employed. After elution is begun, the ratio of the solvents is varied in a programmed way, sometimes continuously and sometimes in a series of steps. Separation efficiency is greatly enhanced by gradient elution.

INSTRUMENTATION OF HPLC

HPLC instrumentation includes a pump, injector, column, detector and integrator or acquisition and display system. The heart of the system is the column where separation occurs.

1. **Solvent Reservoir**: Mobile phase contents are contained in a glass reservoir. The mobile phase, or solvent, in HPLC, is usually a mixture of polar and non-polar liquid components whose respective concentrations are varied depending on the composition of the sample.

2. **Pump**: A pump aspirates the mobile phase from the solvent reservoir and forces it through the system's column and detecter. Depending on a number of factors, including column dimensions, the particle size of the stationary phase, the flow rate and composition of the mobile phase, operating pressures of up to 42000 kPa (about 6000 psi) can be generated.

3. **Sample Injector**: The injector can be a single injection or an automated injection system. An injector for an HPLC system should provide an injection of the liquid sample within the range of 0.1-100 mL of volume with high reproducibility and under high pressure (up to 4000 psi).

4. **Columns**: Columns are usually made of polished stainless steel, are between 50 and 300 mm long and have an internal diameter of between 2 and 5 mm. They are commonly filled with a stationary phase with a particle size of 3–10 μm. Columns with internal diameters of less than 2 mm are often referred to as microbore columns. Ideally, the temperature of the mobile phase and the column should be kept constant during an analysis.

5. **Detector**: The HPLC detector, located at the end of the column, detect the analytes as they elute from the chromatographic column. Commonly used detectors are UV-spectroscopy, fluorescence, mass-spectrometric and electrochemical detectors.

6. **Data Collection Devices**: Signals from the detector may be collected on chart recorders or electronic integrators that vary in complexity and their ability to process, store and reprocess chromatographic data. The computer integrates the response of the detector to each component and places it into a chromatograph that is easy to read and interpret.

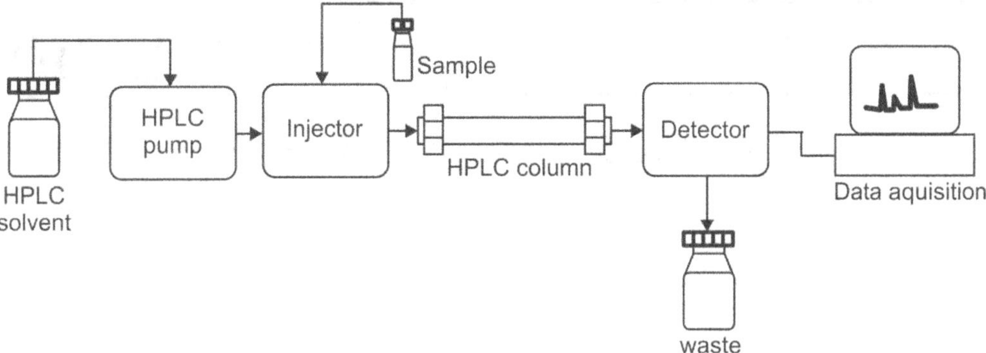

Fig. 7.1 Systematic Diagram of HPLC Instrument.

DETAIL INSTRUMENTATION OF HPLC

- Mobile Phase: Liquid
- Stationary Phase   Separation Mechanism

    - Solid   Adsorption
    - Liquid Layer   Partition
    - Ion exchange resin   Ion exchange
    - Microporous beads   Size Exclusion
    - Chemically modified resin   Affinity

Important Parts of Instrument:

- Solvent Reservoirs
- Pump
- Sample Injector
- Column(s)
- Detector & Data System

Mobile Phase Reservoirs

- Inert containers with inert lines leading to the pump are required.

- Reservoir filters (2-10 mm) at reservoir end of solvent delivery lines

- Degassed solvent

  - Vacuum filtration

  - Sparge with inert gas (N_2 or He)

  - Ultrasonic under vacuum

- Elevate above pumps

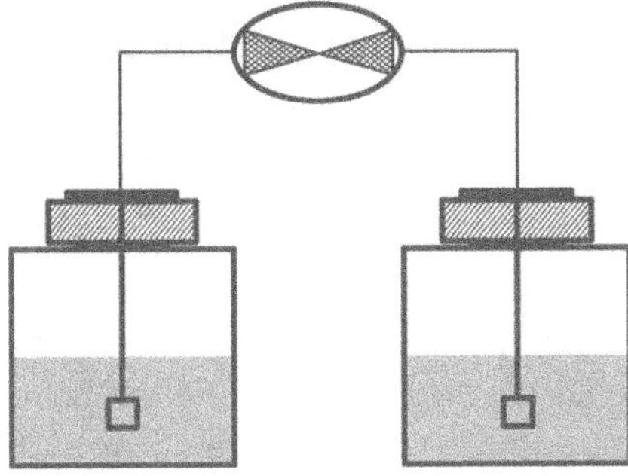

Fig. 8.1 Reservoirs.

Often the reservoirs contain a filtration system for filtering dust and particulate matters from the solvent to prevent these particles from damaging the pumps or injection valves or blocking the column.

The reservoirs are equipped with a degasser for removing dissolved gases- usually oxygen and nitrogen-that interfere by forming bubbles in the column and the detector.

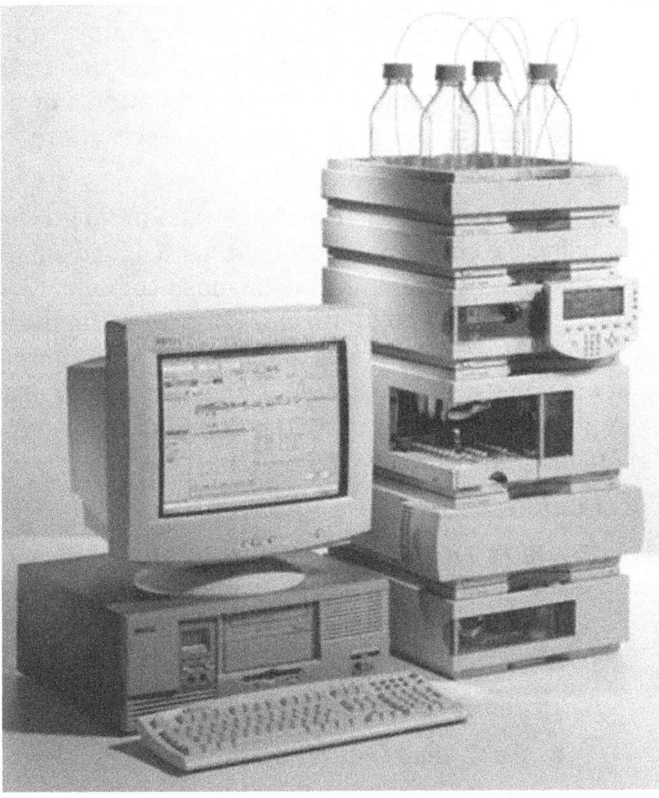

Fig. 8.2 The Agilent 1100, a typical modern LC system.

COLUMN

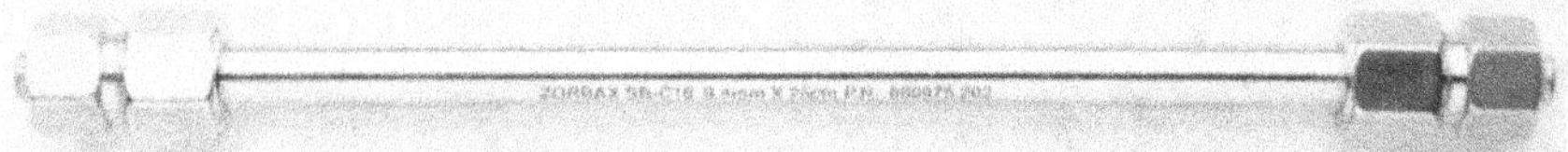

Fig. 8.3 A standard HPLC column.

The stationary phase particles between two trits are held in position by zero dead volume (ZDV) and fittings. The trit porosities may be 2.5 or 10 um, depending upon the particle size of the stationary phase.

A vast majority of the columns used in pharmaceutical industries are made up of stainless steel. Columns made from glass and glass-lined stainless steel are sometimes used for special applications. Less costly stainless steel cartridge columns are often used in quality assurance laboratories. Cartridge columns are essentially tubes packed with stationary phase particles with no end fittings. Reusable holders or end fittings are used to connect the cartridge to the HPLC instrument.

Columns with soft polymer shells are also available commercially. Radially compressed columns, for example, marked by water associates, allow in situ compression of the stationary phase by application of hydraulic pressure to the radius of the column. These columns are cheaper than stainless steel and are available for both analytical and preparative applications.

Liquid-chromatographic columns range in length from 10 to 30 cm. Normally, the columns are straight, with added length, where needed, being gained by coupling two or more columns together. The inside diameter of liquid columns is often 4 to 10 mm; the most common particle size of packings is 5 or 10 µm. The most common column currently in use is one that is 25 cm in length, 4.6 mm inside diameter, and packed with 5 µm particles. Columns of this type contain 40,000 to 60,000 plates/meter

1. **Column Packing**

   The IP (1996) in Appendix 4.3 lists four types of columns which are octadecylsilane (LCI), Octylsilane (LCZ), Porous Silica (LC3), and bonded phase silica (LC4). However, the types of column packing available commercially are very large.

   A. **Types of Column**

   a. **Analytical Columns**

      Liquid-chromatographic columns range in length from 10 to 30 cm. Normally, the columns are straight, with added length, where needed, being gained by coupling two or more columns together. The inside diameter of liquid columns is often 4 to 10 mm; the most common particle size of packings is 5 or 10 μm. The most common column currently in use is one that is 25 cm in length, 4.6 mm inside diameter, and packed with 5 μm particles. Columns of this type contain 40,000 to 60,000 plates/meter.

b. Guard Columns

A guard column is introduced before the analytical column to increase the life of the analytical column by removing not only particulate matter and contaminants from the solvents but also sample components that bind irreversibly to the stationary phase. The guard column serves to saturate the mobile phase with the stationary phase so that losses of this solvent from the analytical column are minimised. The composition of the guard-column packing is similar to that of the analytical column; the particle size is usually larger. When the guard column has become contaminated, it is repacked or discarded and replaced with a new one.

2. Column Length and diameter

For analytical application, the HPLC columns used are 5 cm, 10 cm, 12.5cm, 25cm or 30cm in length and internal diameter (ID) of 3-5 mm.

As a general rule, short analytical columns of 5-15 cm are usually packed with small particles of < 5um. A long column will usually be packed with 10 μm particle size. It will be difficult to pack a long column efficiently with very small particles, e.g. 3um. The backpressure with such columns would be excessive and may not be practical for normal use.

Columns of smaller diameters are often used to reduce solvent consumption. Solvent consumption decrease with the square of the column I.D. Micro and capillary HPLC columns of I.D. less than 1 mm and I.D. of 2 Micro-meter respectively are also available commercially; however, these columns are usually not used routinely for quality control of the drug.

3. Particle Shape and Porosity

Two types of particle shapes are used for packing HPLC columns-Spherical and Irregular. For analytical applications, spherical particles are preferred because these particles are stronger and pack to give reproducible columns. Columns packed with irregular particles initially give efficiency as good as spherical particles, but overused, irregular particles may fracture to give "fines", which may cause a considerable increase in backpressure. Large irregular particles are cheaper and therefore often used for preparative and semi-preparative applications.

The silica-based particles used for the analysis of small molecular weight pharmaceuticals are usually of 6-10 nanometer (nm) pore size. The surface area of the particle may vary from 200-600 m^2g^{-1}.

The particles with a large pore size of 20 nm and above are fragile and have low surface areas. Wide pore size particles are used to analyse large molecular weight compounds such as proteins and polymers.

It is important to note that commercial columns may differ widely among suppliers and were between supposedly identical columns from a single source. The columns can vary in plate number, band asymmetry, retention times, selectivity and lifetimes. The difference in columns with the same functionality, e.g., octdecylsilane, arises from several sources-namely differences in the silica support, choice of silane, monofunctional or polyfunctional, bonding chemistry, pore size, particle size distribution and surface areas of the particles.

4. Derivatisation Column

Derivatisation involves a chemical reaction between an analyte and a reagent to change the chemical and physical properties of an analyte. The four main uses of derivatisation in HPLC are: Improve detectability, change the molecular structure or polarity of the analyte for better chromatography, change the matrix for better separation, and stabilise a sensitive analyte.

Pre or post-primary column derivatisation can be done.

Derivatisation techniques include –acetylation, silylation, and acid hydrolysis.

Disadvantages: It becomes a complex procedure, and so it acts as a source of error to analysis and increases the total analysis time.

Advantages: Although derivatisation has drawbacks, it may still be required to solve a specific separation or detection problem.

5. Fast Column

This column also have the same internal diameter but a much shorter length than most other columns & packed with particles of 3µm in diameter.

Increased sensitivity, decreased analysis time, decreased mobile phase usage & increased reproducibility.

6. Analytical Column

This is the most important part of HPLC, which decides the efficiency of separation

Length- 5 to 25 cm , Internal Diameter 3 to 5mm.

The particle size of the packing material is 3 to 5µm.

LC columns achieve separation by different intermolecular forces b/w the solute & the stationary phase and those b/w the solute & mobile phase.

7. Preparative Column

Length – 10 to 15 cm, Int. diameter – 4.6mm

Packed with particles having 5µm as diameter.

Columns of this time generate 10,000 plates per column.

It consists of a back pressure regulator and fraction collector.

This back pressure regulator is placed posterior to the HPLC detector.

8. Column temperature controller

For obtaining better and reproducible chromatograms, constant column temperature should be maintained.

Some are equipped with heaters that control temperatures to a few tenths of a degree from near ambient.

Columns may also be fitted with water jackets fed from a constant temperature bath to give precise temperature control.

For some applications, close control of column temperature is not necessary & columns are operated at R.T

9. PUMP

The basic requirement of an HPLC pump is that it should deliver the mobile phase through a column at a constant and reproducible flow rate or pressure in a pulse free manner over a long period. The modern HPLC systems have microprocessor controlled pumps which are able to meet the requirements of analysts. Typical analytical HPLC pumps supplied by manufacturers have maximum operating pressures around 5000 bars (7000 psi) and capable of delivering up to 10 ml per min. for analytical HPLC flow rates vary from 0.5-5mlper min. with most applications using flow rates in the range 1-2ml per min.

HPLC Pump Criteria

- Constructed of materials inert toward solvents to be used
- Deliver high volumes (flow rates) of solvent (to 10 mL/min)
- Deliver precise and accurate flow (<0.5% variation)
- Deliver high pressure (to 6000 psi)
- Deliver pulse free flow
- Have low pump-head volume
- Be reliable

HPLC Pumps: Types

- Reciprocating pumps
- Syringe pumps
- Displacement Pump
- Pneumatic Pump
- Constant pressure pumps

10. Reciprocating Pump

The most popular constant flow HPLC pump is the reciprocating pump shown in fig.no.8.4. below

- One, two, or three pump heads
  - more heads, less pulse
- Small head volumes (50 to 250 mL)
- Short piston stroke
- Inert pistons (generally sapphire)
- Continuous use (no refill time)
- Pulse dampeners

Solvent is pumped back and forth by a motor driven piston

Two ball check valves which open & close which controls the flow

The piston is in direct contact with the solvent

Small internal volume 35-400µL

High output pressure up to 10,000 psi

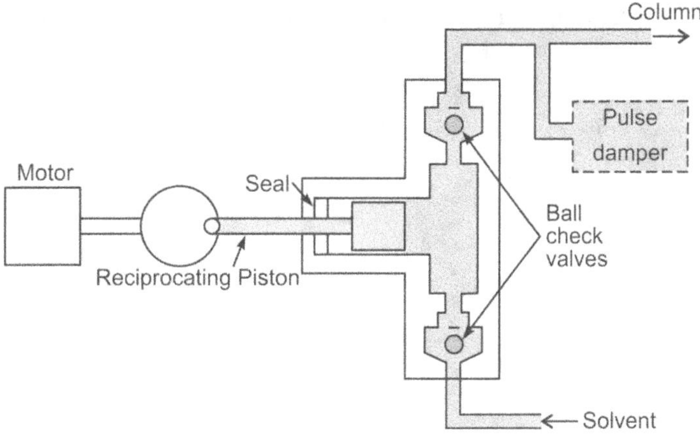

Fig. 8.4 Reciprocating pump.

An eccentric cam drives piston in and out of the solvent chamber. On each forward stroke, the outlet check valve opens and mobile phase is forced in the column, on the return stroke the outlet valve closes and the solvent chamber is filled. The flow rate is changed by varying the length of stroke. In order to obtain pulse less flow, two reciprocating pumps operating at 180⁰ out of phase are used. The pumps have electronics transducers and feed back flow control systems which automatically correct changes in the set flow and out put flow by adjusting the motor speed.

11. Syringe Pump

In syringe type of constant flow pump system, solvent reservoir of 200 to 500 ml capacity is filled with mobile phase.

- Constant flow rate pump
- Non-pulsating flow
- Low flow rates (1 to 100 mL/min)
- Isocratic flow only
- Refill required when reservoir (~50mL) expended

A variable speed stepper motor is used to turn a screw which drives a piston forcing the mobile phase through the column. The flow produced by this type of pump is pulse less. The flow is varied by changing the speed of the motor driving the piston.

12. Displacement Pump

It consists of large, syringe like chambers equipped with a plunger activated by a screw driven mechanism powered by a stepping motor. So it is also called as Screw Driven Syringe Type Pump. It is as shown in Fig 8.5.

Advantages: It produces a flow that tends to be independent of viscosity & back pressure.

Disadvantages: It has a limited solvent capacity(~250) & considerably inconvenient when solvents must be changed

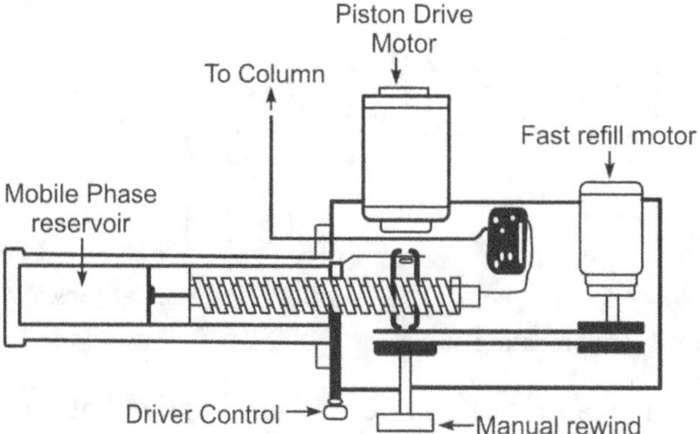

Fig. 8.5 Displacement Pump.

13. Pneumatic Pump

As Shown in Fig. 8.6 in this pump, the mobile phase is driven through the column with the use of pressure produced from a gas cylinder. It has limited capacity of solvent

Due to solvent viscosity back Pressure development.

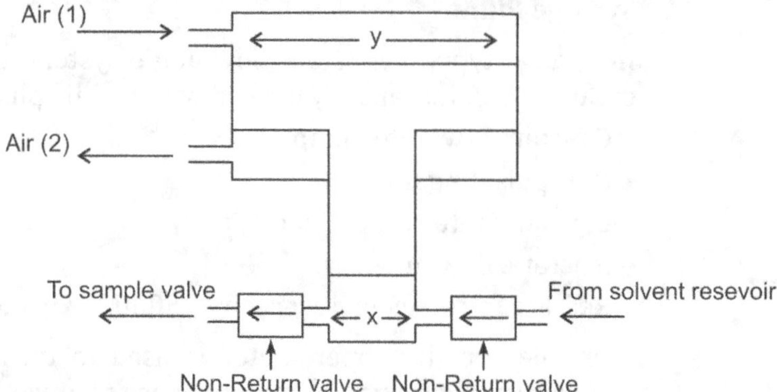

Fig. 8.6 Pneumatic Pump.

14. Constant Pressure Pump

- Constant pressure pump, not constant flow
- Can deliver high pressures
- Stable flow during delivery stroke
- Stop flow on refill stroke
- Low cost

15. Low Pressure and High Pressure Mixing

All manufacturers of the HPLC pumps and systems provide all technical data, mode of operation and limitation of their equipment. However, when purchasing gradient pump one is confronted with two choices- pumps which have low pressure mixing or high pressure mixing of mobile phases.

16. Low pressure mixing

In this type of mixing the arrangement for low pressure mixing pumps of the solvent A & BIn RP-HPLC mobile phases, air bubbles are released when air saturated solvents are mixed. The mixed solvents have a lower capacity for air than pure water or organic solvents such as methanol and acetonitril. The mixture has least capacity for air at intermediate volumes. For pumps using low pressures mixing for gradient run, the problem s most likely to occur near the mid point of the gradient. For low pressure mixing, helium sparing usually reduces the air levels in the solvents to the point at which no out gassing problem persist. In part of India, helium gas may be difficult to obtain on a pump with high. pressure mixing may be the obvious choice.

17. High Pressure Mixing

Fig. 8.7 Shows diagram of the arrangement for high pressure mixing of solvent A & B.

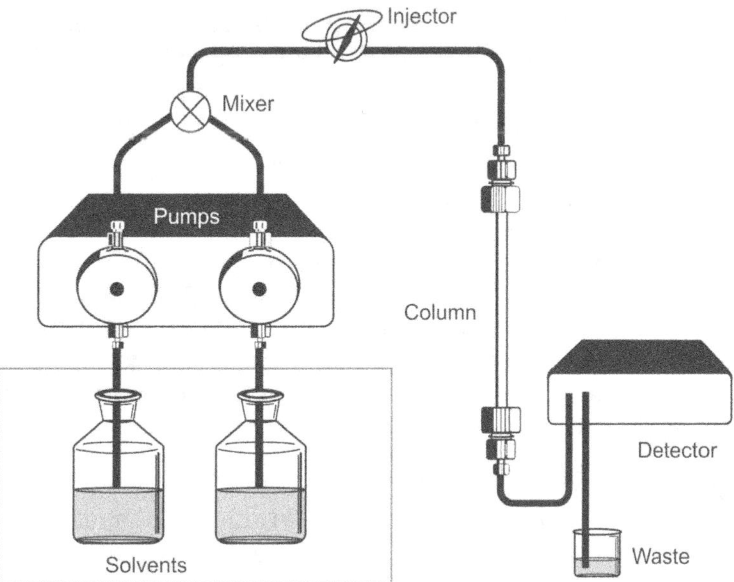

Fig. 8.7 High Pressure Pump.

In case of high pressure mixing, solvents are mixed at high pressure so that air bubbles are kept in solution. When the pressure drops to atmospheric pressure after the mobile phase leaves the detector, the bubbles are released. If bubbles release takes place in or before the detector cell, noise bubbles in the cell may be observed. In most system the release of the pressure can be delayed until after the detector cell by adding a back pressure regulator to the system. This spring loaded regulator mounted on the detector waste line keeps 50-100 psi of back pressure on the system.

18. Isocratic Operation

Both high pressure and low pressure mixing pumps can be used in isocratic mode where only a single solvent is pumped through the column. However problems caused by air bubbles in the mobile phase may present problems. It is therefore advisable to degas the mobile phase either by purging with helium gas for few minutes.

19. Detectors

The function of the detector in HPLC is to monitor the mobile phase emerging from the column. The output of the detector is an electrical signal that is proportional to some property of the mobile phase and for solutes.

Refractive index detector measure the refractive index of both mobile phase and the analyte is called the bulk property detector or universal detector. UV detector or electrochemical detector measure the property possessed essentially by the analyte is called a solute property detector.

20. UV absorbance detector

UV detectors are by far the most popular detectors in HPLC and for pharmaceutical analysis; these detectors are used almost exclusively. Both fixed and variable wavelength uv/visible detector are available. The variable types use a deuterium lamp as a uv radiation source (190nm-400nm) and a tungsten filament (400nm-700nm) for visible range.

The fig. 8.8 show typical UV detector used for HPLC applications.

- **Absorbance Detectors:** Is a Z-shaped, flow-through cell for absorbance measurements on eluents from a chromatographic column. Many absorbance detectors are double-beam devices in which one beam passes through the eluent cell and the other through a filter to reduce its intensity.

- **Ultraviolet Absorbance Detectors with Filters:** The simplest UV absorption detectors are filter photometers with a mercury lamp as the source. Most commonly the intense line at 254 nm is isolated by filters. Deuterium or tungsten filament sources with interference filters also provide a simple means of detecting absorbing species.

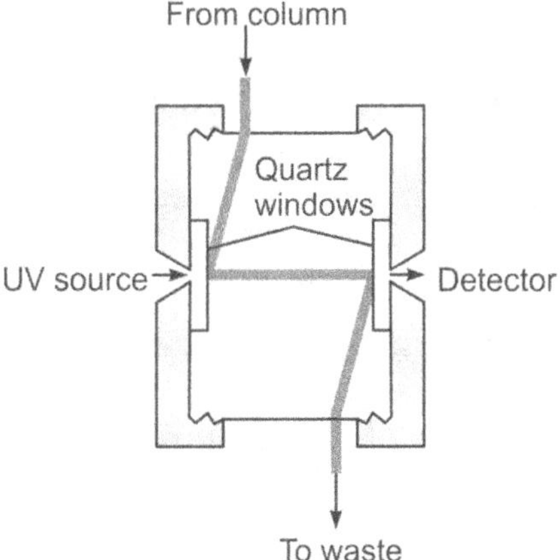

Fig. 8.8 Mode of action of UV detectors.

The absorbance A, of a solution is given by the beer-Lambert law as follows:

$$A= Log[Io/I]=elc$$

Where Io is the intensity of light incident on the sample and I is the transmitted light intensity. Alternatively, A, can also be expressed in trms of analyte concentration, c in the flow cell, analyte molar absorptivity e and flow cell path length l. UV absorbance detectors give an output signal proportional to absorbance rather than transmitted light intensity. The detection wave length and other experimental conditions are selected to maximize the signal equal to absorbance (A) at peak maximum of the sample under examination. The signal aptitude is a function of light path length I of the flow cell. The flow cell is usually 10 mm in length and of approximately 10ul volume.

The fig 3.9 show the same UV source (lamp) transmits light through the sample cell and reference cell. The reference cell is generally inaccessible and therefore usually do not contain solvent. The radiation from the lamp is used as a direct reference beam as the original radiation intensity Io. The electronic system compares the light intensities hitting the two photodiodes and processes the signal into absorption A, which is transmitted to a chart recorder or a computer as an output (A= Log [Io/I]).

Since UV detector is extensively used in HPLC analysis, familiarization of the following parameters for operating a UV detector may prove useful.

21. Operating wavelength

The detection wavelength selected will depend on the UV absorbance of the sample under analysis.

- **UV Absorbance Detector with Monochromator:** There are detectors that consist of a scanning spectrophotometer with grating optics. Some are limited to uv radiation; others encompass both uv and visible radiation. The most powerful uv spectrophotometric detectors are diode-array instruments.

- **Infrared Absorbance Detectors:** Two types of infrared detectors are offered commercially. The range of the first instrument is from 2.5 to 14.5 μm or 4000 to 690 cm^{-1}. The second type of infrared detector is based upon Fourier transform instruments.

The optimum detection wavelength setting is usually the sample UV maximum. Many organic solvents have UV cut off in the region of 220 nm, therefore if a sample has a UV maximum bellow 220nm and a second weak absorbance at longer wavelength, then one may have to select the long wavelength if a suitable organic phase with a UV cut off lower than the peak maximum is not available.

The organic compounds for which UV detectors are of limited application are saturated hydrocarbons. However saturated hydrocarbons substituted by ether (-O-), hydroxyl (-OH), carboxy (-COOH), or ester (-COOR) groups have marginal absorptivuty (ϵ<100) and may require detection at low UV wavelength (190-210nm)

22. Absorbance Range

The range switch of UV detection usually affects the output signal at the chart recorder terminal which may have range of 0-10mV. Most detectors have a second output for computer connection. This is typically 0-1 V range which corresponds to 0-1 absorption unit full scale (a.u.f.s.). 1 a.u.f.s. means that the recorder is registering an absorbance of 1 at full deflection. The output for computer is unaffected by the range switch. Before any analysis is carried out, the detector zero and the recorder zero are synchronized with autozero switch. A autozero will also adjust the detector output to zero volt. The size of the chromatogram appearing on the computer screen is adjusted at the computer itself.

23. Time Constant

The time constant switch (usually located at the back panel of the detector) controls how quickly detector can record a peak. For fast eluting peaks the time constant should not exceed 0.1 second. A very low constant will increase noise and dritt of the detector output signal.

24. Spectral Band Width

The band width of HPLC UV detector is usually of the order of 10 nm. For a wavelength setting of 250nm, for example the radiation covers a range of 255-260nm, that is the filtered light is not monochromatic but covers range within 10 nm. The larger the band width, greater is the light intensity and higher the sensitivity, however if the band width is too wide, the linear range of the output signal may be reduced.

25. The photodiode array detector (PAD)

In the conventional uv / visible detector, polychromatic light is passed through the sample and then focused on to the entrance slit of a monochromator, which passes a narrow band of wavelength to the detector. To obtain spectra, the wavelength is changed by slowly rotating grating in the monochromator. In the PAD (Fig. 8.9) polychromatic radiation, after passing through the sample, is dispersed by a fixed grating and then falls on to an array of photodiodes. Each diode measures a narrow band of wavelengths in the spectrum. The PAD allows parallel data acquisition, all points in the spectrum being measure simultaneously.

The acquisition, processing and storage of spectrum with the PAD detector are fast. A fairly powerful computer is needed to manipulate and store the large amount of data that are generated by the detector. The PAD detector although more expensive than conventional UV detectors are increasingly used for routine analysis. Some of the advantages of the PAD detectors are

a) The spectrum of each peak in the chromatogram can be stored and subsequently compared with standard spectra, which facilitates the identification of peaks

b) The optimum wavelength for single wavelength detection can easily be found

c) Wavelength changes can be programmed to occur at different points in chromatogram to achieve maximum sensitivity for peaks

d) The PDA can provide a counter plot showing the relationship between absorbance, wavelength and time which can be used to detect and identify otherwise unsuspected impurities in the sample.

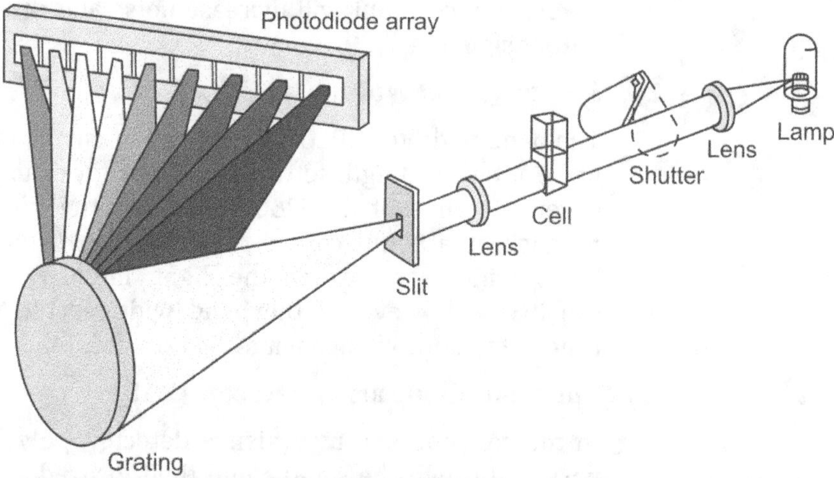

Fig. 8.9 PDA Detector.

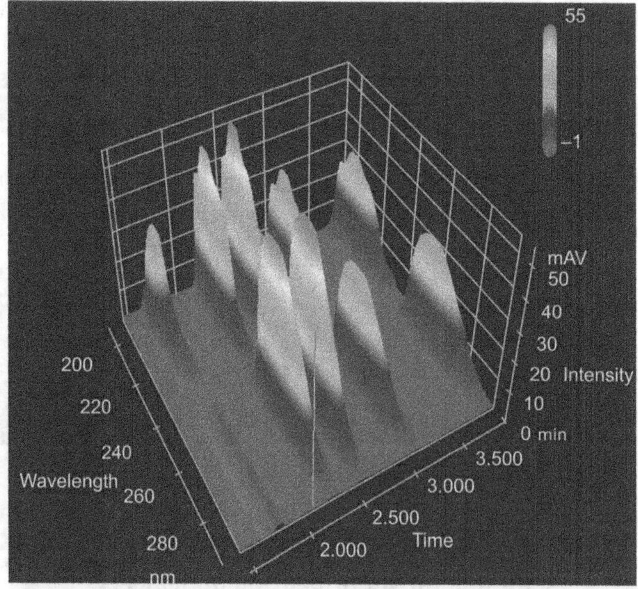

Fig. 8.10 3D Spectra obtained by PDA Detector.

26. Fluorescence Detector

The main attractions of Fluorescence detector in HPLC is that Fluorescence or of which Fluorescing derivatives can be made are detected with high sensitivity and specificity. The sensitivity may be as high as 1000 times greater than with uv detection. The reason for this lies in the difference in the nature of the measurements.

In uv detection, a continuous high intensity of radiation passes through flow cell on to the photo detector. When a chromophore is present, a slight reduction in the radiation occurs. Therefore at high sensitivity, the measurement is one of a very small change in a large signal. In Fluorescence detection, on the other hand, the background radiation signal is almost zero and radiation appears at the photo detector when a fluorescent compound is present.

- Fluorescence is observed by a photoelectric detector located at 90 deg to the excitation beam. The simplest detectors employ a mercury excitation source and one or more filters to isolate a band of emitted radiation. More sophisticated instruments are based upon a Xenon source and employ a grating monochromator to isolate the fluorescent radiation. An inherent advantage of fluorescence methods is their high sensitivity, which is typically greater by more than an order of magnitude than most absorbance procedures.

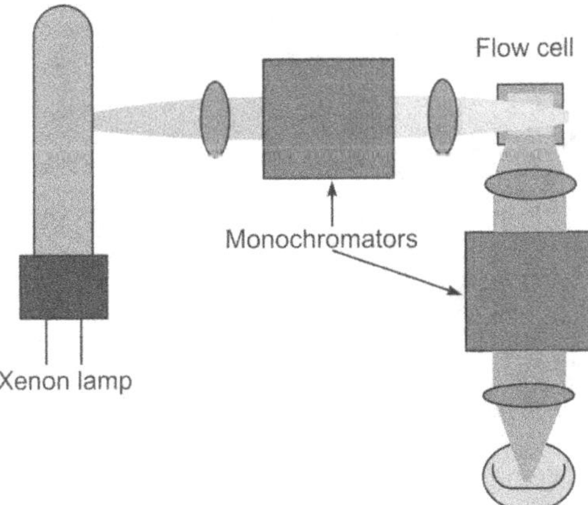

Fig. 8.11 Schematic diagram of Fluorescence detector.

27. Electrochemical Detector

The most commonly used HPLC electrochemical detectors are based on amperometric measurements. The operation of an amperometric detector is based on the oxidation or reduction of sample in a flow through electrolysis cell to which a constant electrical potential is applied. The current from the electrochemical reaction is processed and output for recorder or integrator. The detection limit for compounds which are reduced or oxidized at relatively low potential can be as good as that obtained with fluorescence detector.

These devices are based upon amperometry, polarography, coulometry, and conductometry. They appear to offer advantages, in many instances, of high sensitivity, simplicity, convenience, and widespread applicability.

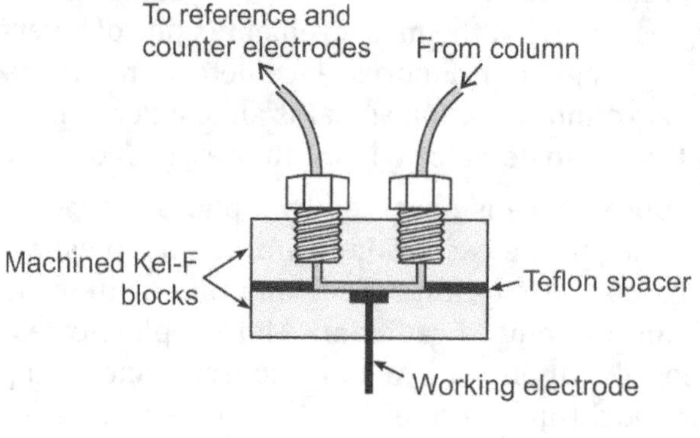

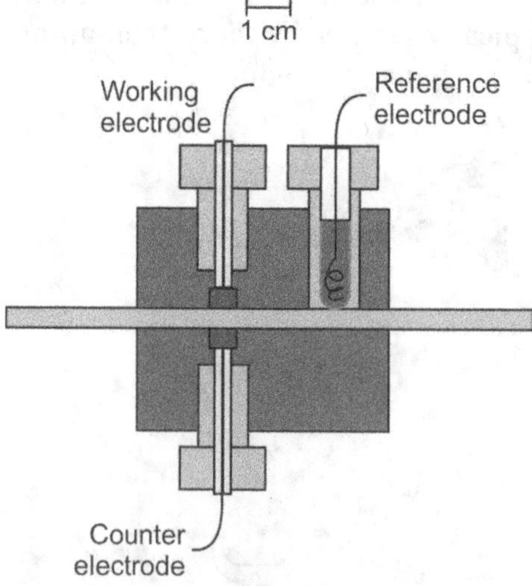

Fig. 8.12 Schematic diagram of Electrochemical detector.

28. Refractive index (RI) detectors

Refractive index (RI) is the ratio of the speed of light in vacuum to that in a given medium. RI is universal property of materials which transmit light. In HPLC, the RI detedtor measure the change in the RI of the mobile phase due to the presence of dissolved sample.

Refractive-index detectors have the significant advantage of responding to nearly all solutes. That is they are general detectors analogous to flame or thermal conductivity detectors in gas chromatography. In addition, they are reliable and unaffected by flow rate. They are, however, highly temperature sensitive and must be maintained at a constant temperature to a few thousandths of a degree centigrade. Furthermore, they are not as sensitive as most other types of detectors.

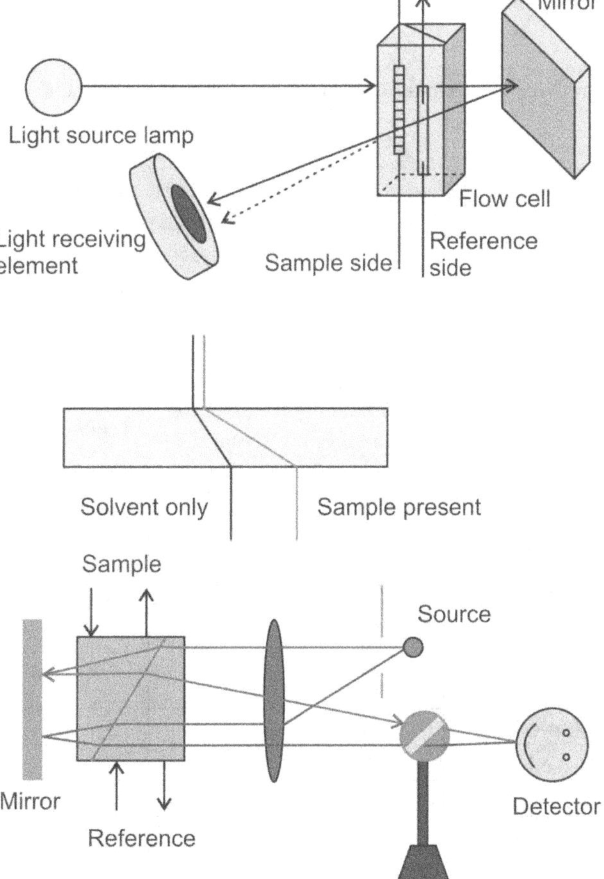

Fig. 8.13 Schematic diagram of Refractive Index detectors.

Table 8.1 Types of Detectors.

Detector	Selectivity	Sensitivity	Notes
Refractive Index	Poor	Poor	Any component that differs in refractive index from the eluate can be detected, despite its low sensitivity. Cannot be used to perform gradient analysis.
UV/Vis	Moderate	Good	A wide variety of substances can be detected that absorb light from 190 to 900 nm. Sensitivity depends strongly on the component.
Fluorescence	Good	Excellent	Components emitting fluorescence can be detected selectively with high sensitivity. This is often used for pre-column and post-column derivatization.
Conductivity	Moderate	Good	Ionized components are detected. This detector is used mainly for ion chromatography.
Electrochemical	Good	Excellent	Electric currents are detected that are generated by electric oxidation-reduction reactions. Electrically active components are detected with high sensitivity.

Table 8.2 Performance of HPLC Detectors.

HPLC Detector	Commercially Available	Mass LOD* (typical)	Linear Range* (decades)
Absorbance	Yes	10 pg	3-4
Fluorescence	Yes	10 fg	5
Electrochemical	Yes	100 pg	4-5
Refractive index	Yes	1 ng	3
Conductivity	Yes	100 pg-1 ng	5
Mass Spectrometry	Yes	<1 pg	5
FTIR	Yes	1 mg	3
Light Scattering	Yes	1 mg	5
Optical Activity	Yes	1 ng	4
Element Selective	Yes	1 ng	4-5
Photoionization	Yes	<1 pg	4

29. Sample Injector

The most popular HPLC Sample Injector is Rheodyne mode 7125 and 7115. 7125 model has an injection port in front of the valve through which sample solution is introduced with a syringe. This valves allows either full loop filling of sample solution. For an externally standardized method full loop filling must be used and minimum of five times the volume of sample is used to fill the loop. E. g. if the loop volume is 20 ul then at least 100 ul of sample solution must be flushed to fill the loop. For an internally standardized method smaller flush volume of the sample may be used.

If the sample available is limited and in cases where it is important that no sample is lost, then partial loop fill may be used i.e. the volume of sample introduced is less than the loop volume.

Several injector devices are available either for manual or auto injection of the sample.

   (i) Septum Injector

   (ii) Stop Flow Injector

   (iii) Rheodyne Injector

- **Valve-type injectors**

   - Six port fixed volume Rheodyne

       reproducible injection volumes

       variable loop size

       easy to use, reliable

   - Six port variable volume Waters

       variable injection volumes without loop change increased maintenance, operator skill require more expensive

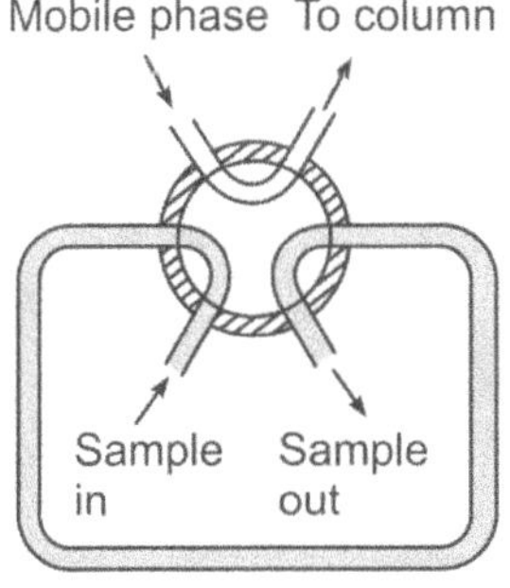

(a) Sampling mode

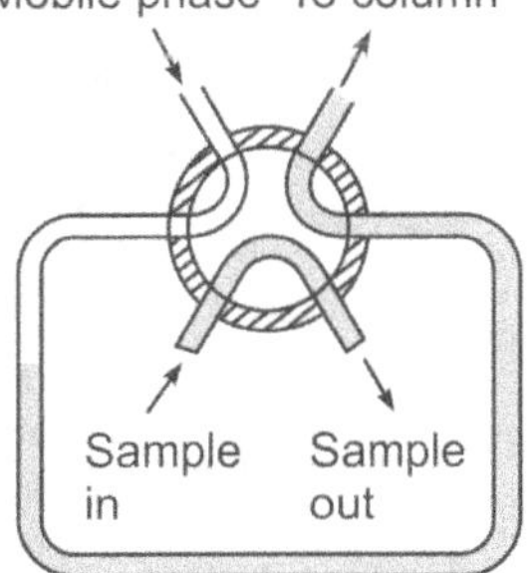

(b) Injection mode

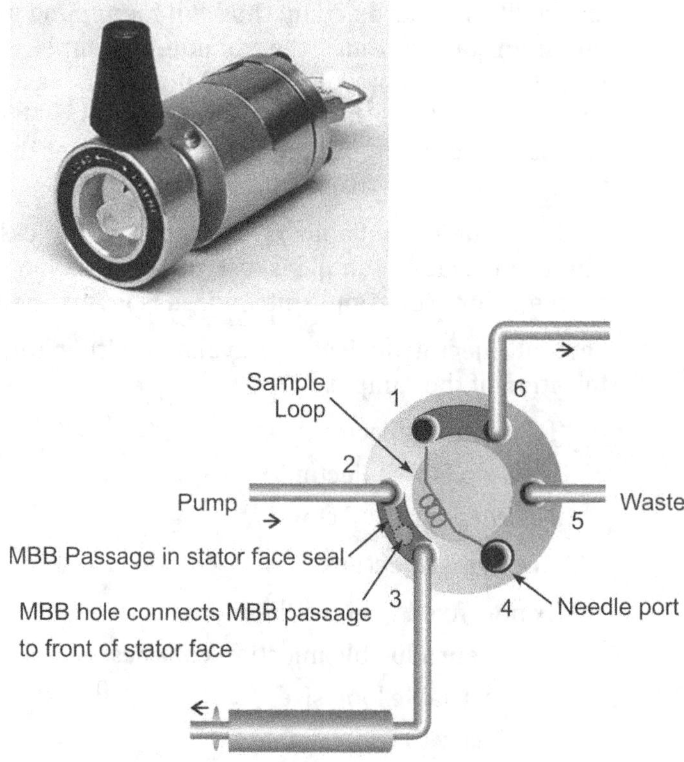

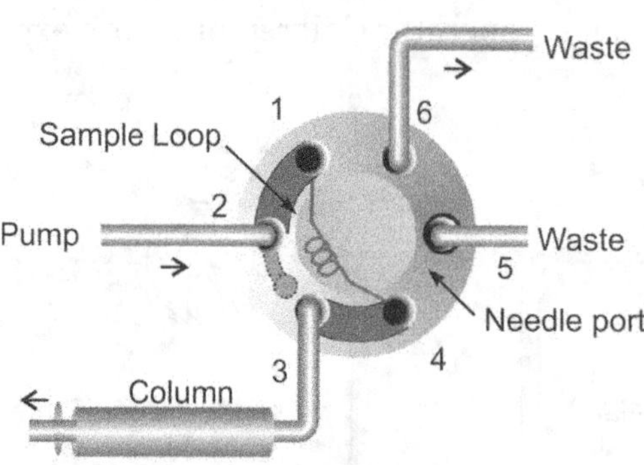

Fig. 8.14 Rheodyne Manual Injector in HPLC.

The Rheodyne Manual Injector is widely used in HPLC. It is the most popular injector and is widely used. This has a fixed volume of loop, for holding sample until its injected into the column, like 20μL, 50μL or more. Through an injector the sample is introduced into the column.The injector is positioned just before the inlet of the column.

30. Auto Injectors

- Continuous injections operator free
- Comparable precision and accuracy to manual
- Much more expensive initially
- Much more convenient Up 100 samples and standards with microprocessor control

31. HPLC Fittings

Standard column end fittings, trits, ferrules, zero dead volume (ZDV) unions and capillary tubing made of stainless steel are marked by almost all supplies of HPLC equipment.

In addition to the standard stainless steel fittings, tubing and column fitting made of polymer polyether ether ketone (PEEK) are also available commercially. PEEK tubes and fittings are resistant to pressure up to 5000 psi. the material is inert to all organic solvents and buffers except concentrated nitric acid, sulphuric acid, tetra hydro furan and methylene chloride.

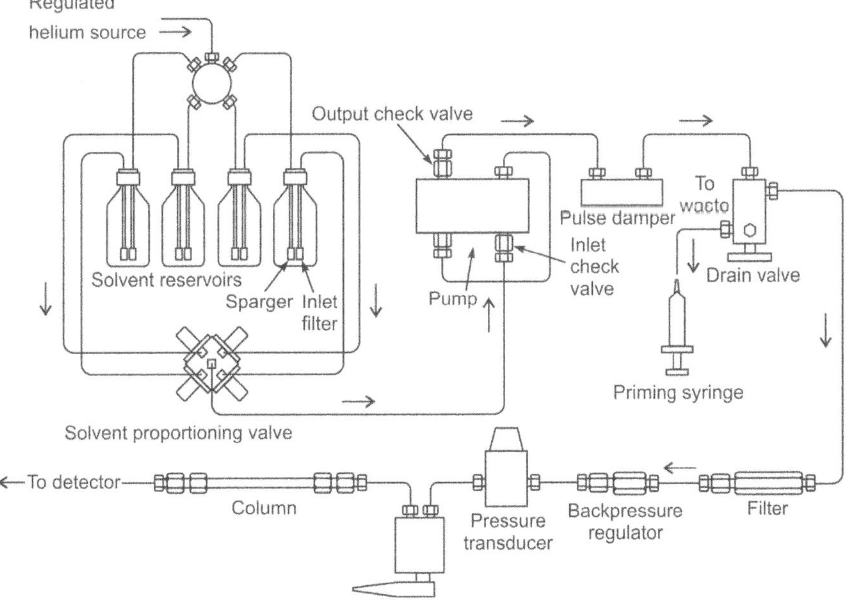

Fig. 8.15 Systemic diagram of HPLC Instrument.

32. Recorders and Integrators

Recorders are used to record responses obtained from the detectors after amplification, if necessary.

They record the baseline & all the peaks obtained with respect tot ime.

Retention time can be found out from this recordings, but area under curve cannot be determined.

33. Integrators

These are improved versions of recorders with some data processing capabilities.

They can record the individual peaks with retention time, height, width of peaks, peak area, percentage area, etc.

Integrators provides more information on peaks than recorders.

In recent days computers and printers are used for recording and processing the obtained data & for controlling several operations.

TYPES OF ELUTION

Elution of solute is carried out by two methods in HPLC as follows.

1. **Isocratic elution:** A separation that employs a single solvent or solvent mixture of constant composition.

2. **Gradient elution:** Here, two or more solvent systems that differ significantly in polarity are employed. After elution is begun, the ratio of the solvents is varied in a programmed way, sometimes continuously and sometimes in a series of steps. Separation efficiency is greatly enhanced by gradient elution.

1. **Isocratic elution:**
   - Isocratic solvents- mobile phase is prepared using pure solvent or mixture of solvents with the same eluting power of polarity.
   - Gradient solvents- in this, the polarity of the solvent is gradually increased & hence the solvent composition has to be changed.

Hence this gradient controller is used when two or more solvent pumps are used for such separations. Simple system with one pump and one solvent reservoir. If more than one solvent is used, solvents should be premixed.

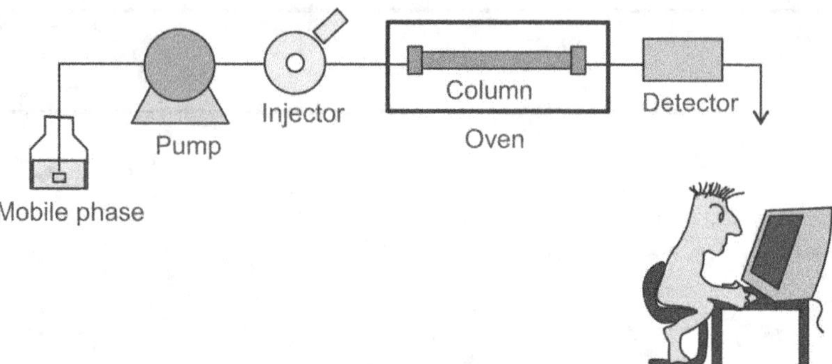

Fig. 9.1 Isocratic Elution System of HPLC.

2.   Gradient elution:

- Excellent gradient accuracy.
- 2-3 pumps required - one pump per solvent used.
- On-line degassing may not be critical

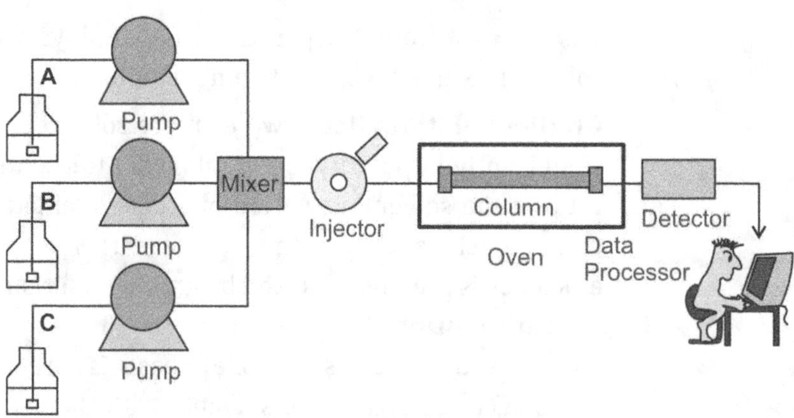

Fig. 9.2 Gradient Elution System of HPLC.

DEGASSING OF SOLVENTS

Several gases are soluble in organic solvents, when high pressure is pumped, the formation of gas bubbles increases which interfere with the separation process, steady baseline & shape of the peak.

Hence de-gassing is very important, and various ways can do it.

(i) Vacuum filtration:

- ✓ De-gassing is accomplished by applying a partial vacuum to the solvent container.
- ✓ But it is not always reliable & complete.

(ii) Helium Purging:
- ✓ Done bypassing Helium
- ✓ Done bypassing Helium through the solvent.
- ✓ This is very effective, but Helium is expensive.

(iii) Ultrasonication:
- ✓ Done by using an ultrasonicator which converts ultra-high-frequency to mechanical vibrations.

CALIBRATION AND VALIDATION (HPLC)

The Calibration of HPLC is carried out as per manual or official standard books, e.g. as per IP

A) Check Liquid Chromatograph (Pump) for the following

    (i) **Checkpoint: Leakage test (By Pressure Drop)**

    (ii) Flow rate calibration

CHECKPOINT: LEAKAGE TEST (BY PRESSURE DROP)

1. Ensure that the instrument is ready for calibration and the Start-up procedure is followed.

2. Place the pump tubing inlet tubing into the Water HPLC grade through the suction filter.

3. Allow the mobile phase to flow for about 5 min.

4. Block Pump outlet with the block screw.

5. The pressure rises, and on crossing the 300 bar, "ERROR P-MAX" appears on the display window. Note the time. Press the "CE" key and observe the pressure drop for 5 min.

6. After 5 min., record the pressure in the calibration Log.

7. Make an entry of the column used in the Column Usage Log Register.

8. Make an entry of the usage into the Instrument Usage Log Register.

9. Compare the result for its compliance against the limit given in the Calibration Log and put the remark regarding the Calibration Status.

10. In case of non-compliance, follow the Maintenance Program.

A-1) Flow rate calibration

1. Ensure that the instrument is ready for calibration and the Start-up procedure is followed.

2. Ensure that the Pump is passing the "Leakage Test (By Pressure Drop)".

3. Keep the Drain tube in such a way that the mobile phase (Water) drops into a 10 ml clean, dry volumetric flask without touching the walls of the flask and start immediately the stopwatch when the first drop falls into the flask.

4. Wait till the collected mobile phase reaches the 10 ml mark of the volumetric flask and Stop the stopwatch.

5. Record the time required to collect the 10 ml mobile phase in the calibration Log.

6. Repeat the procedure for 1.0 ml, 1.5 ml and 2.0 ml/min flow rates.

7. Repeat steps 3 to 6 but use Methanol HPLC grade as mobile phase instead of water.

8. Compare the results for its compliance against limits given in the Calibration Log and put the remark regarding the Calibration Status.

9. Make an entry of the usage of the instrument and column in the Instrument Usage Log Register and Column Usage Log Register, respectively.

10. Prepare the Calibration Status Label and display it on the instrument at the designated place.

11. In case of non-compliance, follow the Maintenance Program.

A-2) Reproducibility and Linearity of Injection Volume

- **Solution Mixer Preparation :**

  1. Take a clean and dry 50 ml volumetric flask.

  2. Pipette out 1.0 ml of Benzene and Toluene into the clean and dry 50 ml volumetric flask.

  3. Make up the volume to 50 ml with Methanol and mix well.

- **Chromatographic Condition :**

Column	:	ODS C18, (25 cm x 4.6 mm ID, 5 µm)
Mobile Phase	:	Methanol : Water (70 : 30)
Flow Rate	:	1.0 ml/min.
Wavelength	:	254 nm
Injection Volume	:	20 µl

Calibration:

1. Ensure that the instrument is ready for calibration and the Start-up procedure is followed.

2. Ensure that the instrument is set according to the Chromatographic conditions.

3. Follow the Instrument Operating procedure, Inject 10 µl in triplicate and record the chromatograms.

4. Repeat the injection of the above solution by injecting 15, 20, 25, and 30 µl in triplicate.

5. Take the printout of the chromatograms and attach it to the Calibration Log.

6. Record the Area and Retention times of the Benzene and Toluene peaks in the Calibration Log.

7. Make an entry of the usage of the instrument and column in the Instrument Usage Log Register and Column Usage Log Register, respectively.

8. Plot the curve for the area corresponding to Benzene to Toluene peaks v/s injection volume; find out the RSD (reproducibility) and record it in the Calibration Log.

9. Find out the Correlation coefficient "r^2" for each peak at five levels and record it in the Calibration Log.

10. Compare the result for its compliance against the limit given in the Calibration Log and put the remark regarding the Calibration Status.

11. Prepare the Calibration Status Label and display it on the instrument at the designated place.

12. In case of non-compliance, follow the Maintenance Program.

B) Check the Liquid Chromatograph (UV Detector) for the following:

Checkpoint: D_2 Lamp Energy Check (Detector)

1. Ensure that the instrument is ready for calibration and the Start-up procedure is followed.

2. On the Detector's display window, some values at the functions "l(nm)", "abs(AU)", "range(AUFS)", and "lamp" appear.

3. On the display, the previously set value blinks at "l(nm)" function; enter the Wavelength to 254 nm by pressing numerical keys.

4. Press the "Func Back" key and select "lamp" functions; enter 1 to select D_2 lamp.

5. Further press "Func Back" key till "REF EN " appears.

6. Record the Reference Energy of the D2 Lamp at 254 nm in the Calibration Log.

7. Compare the result for its compliance against the limit given in the Calibration Log and put the remark regarding the Calibration Status.

8. In case of non-compliance, follow the Maintenance Program.

B-1)   Linearity of Detector Response:

- **Solution Mixer Preparation :**

    1. Take three clean and dry 50 ml volumetric flasks.

    2. Pipette out ml of Benzene and Toluene as per the following table into the clean, dry 50 ml volumetric flask separately.

    3. Make up the volume to 50 ml with Methanol and mix well.

Table 10.1 Readings of Linearity

Solution (Level)	ml of Benzene to be taken	Ml of Toluene to be taken	To be Diluted with Methanol to
1	0.5	1.0	50 ml
2	1.0	1.0	50 ml
3	1.5	1.0	50 ml

- **Chromatographic Condition :**

    1. **Set each equipment to the following parameters as per the Equipment's Parameter Set Up Procedure.**

Column	:	ODS C18, (25 cm x 4.6 mm ID, 5 m)
Mobile Phase	:	Methanol : Water (70 : 30)
Flow Rate	:	1.0 ml/min.
Wavelength	:	254 nm
Injection Volume	:	20 µl

Calibration:

1. Ensure that the instrument is ready for calibration and the Start-up procedure is followed.

2. Ensure that the instrument is set according to the Chromatographic conditions.

3. Follow the Instrument Operating procedure, Inject each of the Solutions in triplicate and record the chromatograms.

4. Take the printout of the chromatograms and attach it to the Calibration Log.

5. Record the Area and Retention times of the Benzene and Toluene peaks in the Calibration Log.

6. Make an entry of the usage of the instrument and column in the Instrument Usage Log Register and Column Usage Log Register, respectively.

7. Calculate the Area Ratio of Benzene to Toluene, Find out the Mean value of the ratios and record it in the Calibration Log.

8. Find out the Correlation coefficient "r^2" from the Mean area ratio values of the three levels. Record in the Calibration Log.

9. Plot the curve for area ratio corresponding to Benzene to Toluene peaks v/s concentration; find out the RSD (reproducibility) and record it in the Calibration Log.

10. Compare the result for its compliance against the limit given in the Calibration Log and put the remark regarding the Calibration Status.

11. Prepare the Calibration Status Label and display it on the instrument at the designated place.

12. In case of non-compliance, follow the Maintenance Program.

Table 10.2 Calibration of HPLC Pump

Model No.   :   Make   :

Instrument Code No.   :

A. Check point : Leakage Check Test (Pressure Drop)						
P.Max to be set	P.Max Set	Start Time	Stop Time	Total Time	Pressure Observed	Remark
300 bar						
B. Flow Rate calibration :						
Flow Rate (ml/min)	Time required to collect 10 ml mobile phase			Limit	Remarks	
	Theoretical (in sec.)	Actual with water	Actual with Methanol			
0.5 ml	1200			1194 - 1206		
1.0 ml	600			594 – 606		
1.5 ml	450			443 – 457		
2.0 ml	300			294 - 306		

Calibration Status   : Satisfactory / Not Satisfactory

Next Calibration Due   :

Calibrated By   :   Checked By   :

Date   :   Date   :

Table 10.3 Calibration Of Injector

Model　　　　　　　:　　　　　　　　　　Make　　　　:

Instrument Code No.　:

a. Preparation of solvent mixture :

Taken ____ ml (1.0 ml) of the ______ (Benzene) and ______ (Toluene) in to a ____ ml (50 ml) clean, dry volumetric flask, make up the volume with methanol, mixed well.

B. Chromatographic Condition :

Parameters	*Test Condition*	*Applied Condition*
Mobile Phase	Methanol: Water (70 : 30)	
Column	**ODS C18, (25 cm x 4.6 mm ID, 5 μm)**	
Flow Rate	*1.0 ml / min.*	
Wavelength	*254 nm*	

Injection volume		*Injection -1*		*Injection -2*		*Injection -3*		*Mean*	*% RSD : (Not more than 2.0%)*
		Benzene	*Toluene*	*Benzene*	*Toluene*	*Benzene*	*Toluene*		
10 ml	*RT*								
	Area								
15 ml	*RT*								
	Area								
20 ml	*RT*								
	Area								
25 ml	*RT*								
	Area								
30 ml	*RT*								
	Area								

Coefficient of co relations : r^2 : __________ (Limit : NLT : 0.999)

Calibration Status　　: Satisfactory / Not Satisfactory

Next Calibration Due　:

Calibrated By:　　　　　　　　　　　　　　Checked By　:

Date　　　:　　　　　　　　　　　　　　　Date　　:

Fig. 10.1 Calibration of Detector.

Model   :   Make   :

Instrument Code No.   :

D2 LAMP ENERGY CHECK :			
Wavelength to be set	Wavelength Set	Reference Energy Observed	Limit
254 nm			Not less than 200

LINEARITY OF DETECTOR RESPONSE :						
a. Solution Preparation :						
Solution	ml of Benzene		ml of Toluene		in Methanol	
(Level)	To be taken	Taken	To be taken	Taken	To be diluted	Diluted to
1	0.5 ml		1.0 ml		50 ml	
2	1.0 ml		1.0 ml		50 ml	
3	1.5 ml		1.0 ml		50 ml	

Mobile Phase Preparation : Taken _____ ml of _________ (Methanol HPLC grade) in to a ______ ml clean, dry volumetric flask, added _________ ml of _________(Water HPLC grade), mixed well, allowed to cool to room temperature. Filtered through 0.45/0.22 m membrane filter, degassed for _____ min. by vacuum / sonication.

Parameters	Test Condition	Applied Condition
Mobile Phase	Methanol : Water (70 : 30)	
Column	ODS C18, (25 cm x 4.6 mm ID, 5 μm)	
Flow Rate	1.0 ml / min.	
Wavelength	254 nm	
Range	1.0 AUFS	
Injection Volume	20 μl	

Solution	Benzene Area		Toluene Area		Area Ratio
(Level)	RT	Area	RT	Area	(Benzene/Toluene)
1					
Mean :					
% RSD :		---		---	

Table *Contd…*

2					
Mean :					
% RSD :					
3					
Mean :					
% RSD :					

Linearity of Ratio : Correlation Co-efficient r^2 :
Limit : % RSD of the Retention Time : Not more than 2.0%
Linearity of Ratio : Correlation Co-efficient r^2 : Not less than 0.999

Calibration Status   : Satisfactory / Not Satisfactory

Next Calibration Due   :

Calibrated By   :   Checked By   :

Date   :   Date   :

ELEVEN

NEW METHOD DEVELOPMENT & VALIDATION AS PER ICH GUIDELINES

BASIC STEPS INVOLVED IN METHOD DEVELOPMENT OF HPLC

The basic requirement for any new method development by HPLC is to use spectroscopy to select solvent & λ_{max}.

Most drugs in their formulations can be analysed by spectrophotometric methods. Because it is an easy, accurate, fast, and economical method for estimating colourless and coloured components. It is a very old and basic technique for estimating the known component and also guesses functional groups in unknown compounds. Absorption spectra were obtained as per functional groups present in the compound. The colourless drug components were scanned to 200-400 nm and coloured at 400-800 nm visible range. The wavelength is fixed when the drug component shows maximum absorbance (λ_{max}). Nowadays, HPLC is commonly used for the estimation of multicomponent drugs and plays an important role in the estimation of pure drugs and formulation in quality control and quality assurance.

Spectroscopic measurement depends on the following conditions like,

- solvents used,
- wavelength selected and
- Selection of HPLC system

Selection of Solvent

The solute should be completely soluble in the respective solvent. In UV detection, the wavelength of the solvent should not interfere with the absorbance of the drug component, and the solution of drugs should be stable at room temperature. Commonly water, a mixture of organic solvents and water, is used as the solvent.

Selection of Wavelength

The sensitivity of UV absorption depends upon the proper selection of the wavelength. An ideal wavelength gives a good response for all the components to be detected. However, this may not be possible in all cases due to the difference in the nature of the drugs present in the multicomponent dosage forms.

UV spectrums of 10 µg/ml of standard drugs were recorded individually. The spectrums were superimposed to get an overlay spectrum for two or three drugs as per combination in the formulation. From this overlain spectrum, detection wavelength was fixed at which all the drugs show good absorbance.

The selection of different wavelengths depends upon λ_{max} obtained for different drug components and overlay spectrum for multicomponent drugs. If the drug components are not giving better absorbance, then derivatisation of spectra taken for selection of wavelength.

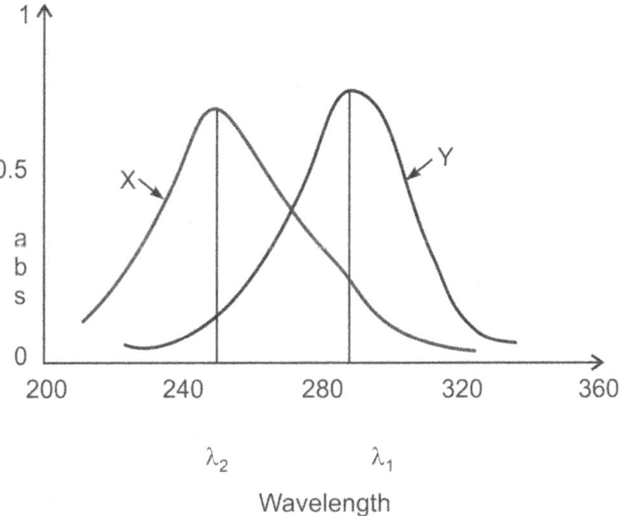

Fig. 11.1 The individual absorption spectra of drugs X and Y, showing the Overlay of two drugs.

Selection of wavelength for HPLC Method development is the maximum absorbance of the individual drug as well as separation of peaks distinctly, The retention time RT of each drug molecule should be separate and within 20 mins RT.

1.   Estimation of multi component dosage forms by HPLC

Most of the drugs in multicomponent dosage forms can be analysed by the HPLC method because of several advantages like rapidity, specificity, accuracy, precision, and ease of automation. HPLC method eliminates tedious extraction and isolation procedures. Some of the advantages are,

- Speed (analysis can be accomplished in 20 minutes or less),
- Greater sensitivity (various detectors can be employed),
- Improved resolution (wide variety of stationary phases)
- Reusable columns (expensive columns but can be used for many analysis),
- Ideal for substances of low volatility,
- Easy sample recovery, handling and maintenance,
- Instrumentation lends itself to automation and quantitation (less time and labour),
- Precise and reproducible,
- Calculations are done by the integrator itself and
- Suitable for preparative liquid chromatography on a much larger scale.

There are different modes of separation in HPLC. Normal phase mode, reverse phase mode, reverse phase ion pair chromatography, ion-exchange chromatography, affinity chromatography and size exclusion chromatography (gel permeation and gel filtration chromatography).

In the normal phase mode, the stationary phase is polar, and the mobile phase is non-polar in nature. In this technique, non-polar compounds travel faster and are eluted first. This is because of the lower affinity between the non-polar compounds and the stationary phase. Polar compounds are retained for longer times because of their higher affinity with the stationary phase. These compounds, therefore, take more time to elute. Normal phase mode of separation is, therefore, not generally used for pharmaceutical applications because most of the drug molecules are polar in nature and hence take a longer time to elute.

The reverse-phase mode is the most popular mode for analytical and preparative separations of the compound of interest in chemical, biological, pharmaceutical, food and biomedical sciences. In this mode, the stationary phase is a non-polar hydrophobic packing with an octyl or octadecyl functional group bonded to silica gel, and the mobile phase is a polar solvent. An aqueous mobile phase allows the use of secondary solute chemical equilibrium (such as ionisation control, ion suppression, ion-pairing and complexation) to control retention and selectivity. The polar compound gets eluted first in this mode, and non polar compounds are retained for a longer time. As most of the drugs and pharmaceuticals are polar in nature, they are not retained for longer times and hence elute faster. The different columns used are octadecyl silane (ODS) or C18, C8, C4 etc. (in the order of increasing polarity of the stationary phase).

In ion-exchange chromatography, the stationary phase contains ionic groups like NR3+ or SO3-, which interact with ionic groups of the sample molecules. This is suitable for the separation of charged molecules only. Changing the pH and salt concentration can modulate the retention.

Ion pair chromatography may be used for the separation of ionic compounds, and this method can also substitute for ion-exchange chromatography. Strong acidic and basic compounds may be separated by reverse-phase mode by forming ion pairs (columbic association species formed between two ions of opposite electrical charge) with suitable counterions. The technique is referred to as reverse phase ion pair chromatography or soap chromatography.

Affinity chromatography uses highly specific biochemical interactions for separations. The stationary phase contains specific groups of molecules which can absorb the sample if certain stearic and charge related conditions are satisfied. This technique can be used to isolate proteins, enzymes, as well as antibodies from a complex mixture.

Size exclusion chromatography separates molecules according to their molecular mass. The largest molecules are eluted first, and the smallest molecules last. This method is generally used when a mixture contains compounds with at least a 10% molecular mass difference. This mode can be further subdivided into gel permeation chromatography (with organic solvent) and gel filtration chromatography (with aqueous solvents).

The various components of HPLC are pumps (solvent delivery system), mixing unit, gradient controller and solvent degasser, injector (manual or auto), guard column, analytical columns, detectors, recorders and /or integrators. Recent models are equipped with computers and software for data acquisition and processing.

The choice of the column should be made after careful consideration of the mode of the chromatographic technique. Three columns are available based on the type of packing and particle size, namely, rigid solids, hard gels, and porous and pellicular layer beads. The columns of smaller particles (3-10 µ) are always preferred because they offer high efficiency (number of theoretical plates/meter) and speed of analysis.

The different types of detection used in HPLC methods are ultraviolet (UV) detection, fluorescence detection, refractive index detection, mass spectrophotometric detection and electrochemical detection. In most cases, method development in HPLC is carried out with UV detection using a variable wavelength spectrophotometric detector or a diode array detector (DAD).

Digital electronic integrators are widely used today in HPLC for measuring peak areas. These devices automatically sense peaks and print out the areas in numerical form. Computing integrators are even more sophisticated and offer a number of features in addition to basic digital integration because these devices have both memory and computing capabilities to upgrade integrating parameters to maintain accuracy as the separation progress and eluting peaks become broader. Many of these devices print out a complete report, including names of the compounds, retention times, and peak areas correction factors. With the help of peak area and height values, the peak width can be used to calculate the number of theoretical plates.

2. Method development and design of separation method by HPLC

Methods for analysing drugs in multicomponent dosage forms can be developed, provided one has knowledge about the nature of the sample, namely, its molecular weight, polarity, ionic character and solubility parameter. However, an exact recipe for HPLC cannot be provided because method development involves considerable trial and error procedures. The most difficult problem usually is where to start, what type of column is worth trying with what kind of mobile phase. In general, one being with reverse phase chromatography when the compounds are hydrophilic in nature with many polar groups and are water-soluble.

The organic phase concentration required for the mobile phase can be estimated by the gradient elution method. The best way to start is with gradient reverse phase chromatography for aqueous sample mixtures. Gradients can be started with a 5-10% organic phase in the mobile phase, and the organic phase concentration (methanol or acetonitrile) can be increased up to 100% within 30-45 min. Separation can be optimised by changing the initial mobile phase composition and slope of the gradient according to the chromatogram obtained from the preliminary run. The initial mobile phase composition can be estimated based on where the compounds of interest were eluted, namely, at what mobile phase composition.

The elution of drug molecules can be altered by changing the polarity of the mobile phase. The elution strength of a mobile phase depends upon its polarity, the stronger the polarity, the higher is the elution. Ionic samples (acidic or basic) can be separated if they are present in the undissociated form. Dissociation of ionic samples may be suppressed by the proper selection of pH.

The pH of the mobile phase has to be selected in such a way that the compounds are not ionised. If the retention times are too short, the decrease of the organic phase concentration in the mobile phase can be in steps of 5%. If the retention times are too long, an increase in the organic phase concentration is needed.

In UV detection, good analytical results are obtained only when the wavelength is selected carefully. This requires knowledge of the UV spectra of the individual components present in the sample. If analyte standards are available, their UV spectra can be measured prior to HPLC method development.

The molar absorbance at the detection wavelength is also an important parameter. When peaks are not detected in the chromatograms, it is possible that the sample quantity is not enough for the detection. An injection of a volume of 20 µl from a solution of 1 mg/ml concentration normally provides good signals for UV active compounds around 220 nm. Even if the compounds exhibit higher λ_{max}, they absorb strongly at a lower wavelength. It is not always necessary to detect compounds at their maximum absorbance. It is, however, advantageous to avoid the detection at the sloppy part of the spectrum for precise quantisation. When acceptable peaks are detected on the chromatogram, the investigation of the peak shapes can help further method development.

The addition of a peak modifier to the mobile phase can affect the separation of ionic samples. For example, the retention of the basic compounds can be influenced by the addition of small amounts of triethylamine (a peak modifier) to the mobile phase. Similarly, a small amount of acetic acid can be used for acidic compounds. This can lead to useful changes in selectivity.

When tailing or fronting is observed, it means that the mobile phase is not totally compatible with the solutes. In most cases, the pH is not properly selected, and hence partial dissociation or protonation takes place. If peak shape does not improve by using lower (1-2) or higher (8-9) pH, then ion-pair chromatography can be used. For acidic compounds, cationic ion pair molecules at higher pH, and for basic compounds, anionic ion pair molecules at lower pH can be used. For amphoteric solutes or a mixture of acidic and basic compounds, ion-pair chromatography is the method of choice.

The low solubility of the sample in the mobile phase can also cause bad peak shapes. It is always advisable to use the same solvent to prepare the sample solution as the mobile phase to avoid precipitation of the compounds in the column or injector.

Optimisation can be started only after a reasonable chromatogram has been obtained. A reasonable chromatogram means that all the compounds are detected by more or less symmetrical peaks on the chromatogram. By a slight change in the mobile phase composition, the shifting of the peaks can be expected. From a few experimental measurements, the position of the peak can be predicted within the range of investigated changes. An optimised chromatogram is one in which all the peaks are symmetrical and are well separated in less run time.

The peak resolution can be increased by using a more efficient column (column with a higher theoretical plate number, N) which can be achieved by using a column of smaller particle size or a longer column. These factors, however, will increase the analysis time. Flow rate does not influence resolution, but it has a strong effect on the analysis time.

The parameters that are affected by the changes in chromatographic conditions are,

- Retention time (Rt)
- Resolution (Rs),
- Capacity factor (k'),
- Selectivity (α),
- Column efficiency (N) and
- Peak asymmetry factor (As)

2. Quantitative analysis in HPLC

Three methods are generally used for quantitative analysis. They are the external standard method, the internal standard method and the standard addition method.

(i) External standard method

The external method involves the use of a single standard or up to three standard solutions. The peak area or the height of the sample and the standard used are compared directly. One can also use the slope of the calibration curve based on standards that contain known concentrations of the compounds of interest.

(ii) Internal standard method

A widely used technique of quantitation involves the addition of an internal standard to compensate for various analytical errors. In this approach, a known compound of a fixed concentration is added to the known amount of samples to give separate peaks in the chromatograms to compensate for the losses of the compounds of interest during sample pretreatment steps. Any loss of the component of interest will be accompanied by the loss of an equivalent fraction of the internal standard. The accuracy of this approach obviously depends on the structural equivalence of the compounds of interest and the internal standard.

The requirements for an internal standard are,

- it must have a completely resolved peak with no interferences,
- it must elute close to the compound of interest,
- it must behave equivalent to the compounds of interest for
- analysis like pretreatments, derivative formations, etc.,
- it must be added at a concentration that will produce a peak area or peak height ratio of about unity with the compounds of interest,
- it must not be present in the original sample,
- it must be stable, unreactive with sample components, column packing & the mobile phase and
- it is desirable that the compound is commercially available in high purity.

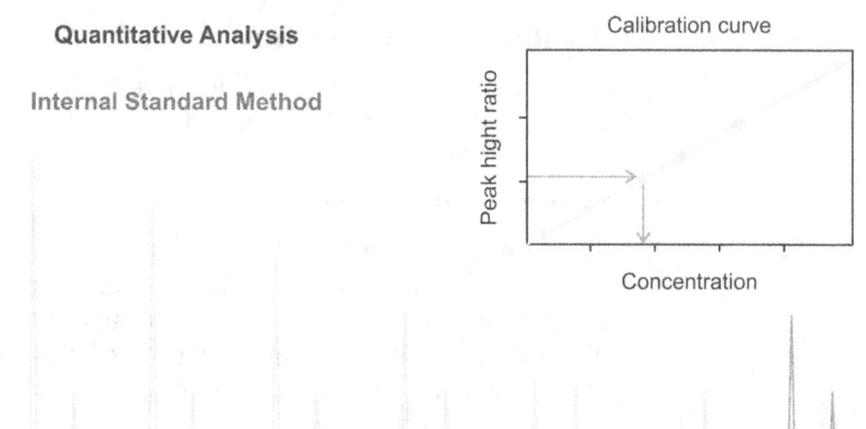

Fig. 11.2 Internal Standard method.

The internal standard should be added to the sample prior to the sample preparation procedure and homogenised with it. To recalculate the concentration of a sample component in the original sample, one has to first determine the response factor. The response factor (RF) is the ratio of peak areas of the sample component (Ax) and the internal standard (AISTD) obtained by injecting the same quantity. It can be calculated using the formula,

$$RF = Ax / AISTD$$

When more than one component is to be analysed from the same sample, the response factor of each component should be determined.

(iii) Standard addition method

In the standard addition method, a known amount of the standard compound is added to the sample solution to be estimated. This method is suitable if a sufficient amount of the sample is available and is more realistic in the sense that it allows calibration in the presence of excipients or other components.

TWELVE

VALIDATION OF NEW HPLC METHOD DEVELOPED AS PER ICH GUIDELINES

Validation is a process that confirmation or establishment by laboratory studies that a method developed is accurate, precise and rugged. In simple terms, validation of an analytical procedure is to demonstrate that the procedure developed is suitable for its intended purpose and it works in a reproducible manner when carried out by the same or different persons, in the same or different laboratories, using different brands of reagents and equipment, etc.,

The various validation performance parameters are,

- accuracy,
- precision (repeatability and reproducibility),
- specificity,
- linearity and range,
- limit of detection (LOD)/limit of quantization (LOQ),
- selectivity/specificity,
- ruggedness/robustness,
- stability and
- system suitability.

ACCURACY

The accuracy of an analytical method is the closeness of test results obtained by that method to the true value. The accuracy of an analytical method should be established across its range. Accuracy is calculated as the percentage of recovery by the assay of the known added amount of analyte in the sample, or as the difference between the mean and the accepted true value, together with confidence intervals.

Accuracy is calculated from the test results as the percentage of analyte recovered by the assay. Dosage form assays commonly provide accuracy within 3-5% of the true value.

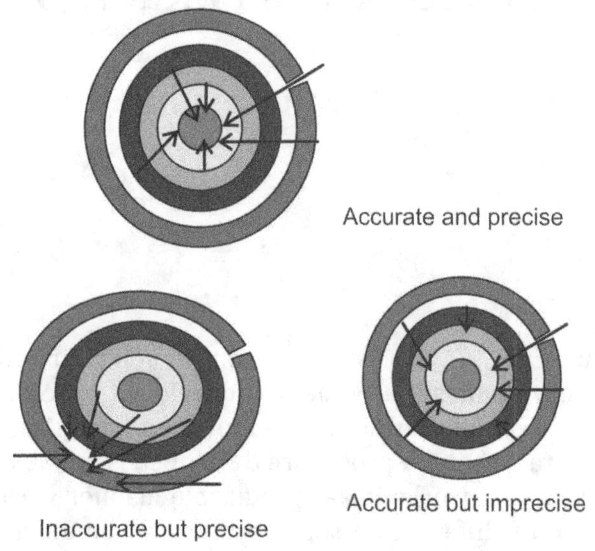

Fig. 12.1 Accuracy & Precision.

PRECISION

The precision of an analytical method is the degree of agreement among individual test results when the method is applied repeatedly to multiple samplings of a homogeneous sample. The precision of an analytical method is usually expressed as the standard deviation or relative standard deviation (coefficient of variation) of a series of measurements. The precision of an analytical method is determined by assaying a sufficient number of aliquots of a homogeneous sample to be able to calculate statistically valid estimate of standard deviation or relative standard deviation. The precision determinations permit an estimate of the reliability of a single determination and are commonly in the range of 0.3 to 3% for dosage form assays.

SPECIFICITY

The International Conference of Harmonization (ICH) documents define specificity as the ability to assess the analyte unequivocally in the presence of components that may be expected to be present, such as impurities, degradation products and matrix components.

In the case of an assay, demonstration of specificity requires that the procedure is unaffected by the presence of impurities or excipients. In practice, it can be done by spiking the substance or product with appropriate levels of impurity or recipients and demonstrating that the assay results are unaffected by the presence of this extraneous material.

If impurity or degradation product standards are unavailable, specificity may be demonstrated by comparing test results of samples containing impurities or degradation products to a well-characterized procedure. This comparison should include sample stored under relevant stress conditions, e.g., light, heat, humidity, acid/base hydrolysis and oxidation.

SELECTIVITY

The selectivity of an analytical method is its ability to measure accurately and specifically the analyte of interest in the presence of components that may be expected to be present in the same matrix. Selectivity in HPLC is usually expressed by the minimum resolution factor (Rs) of two neighbouring peaks and peak purity. The peak purity can be checked by subtracting two chromatograms of the sample obtained at two different wavelengths. If the peak is pure, the absorption ratio at the two wavelengths should be exactly the same from the beginning to the end of the peak.

The selectivity of the analytical method is determined by comparing test results from the analyses of samples containing impurities or degradation products or placebo ingredients with those obtained from the analyses of samples without impurities or degradation products or placebo ingredients.

LINEARITY AND RANGE

The linearity of an analytical method is its ability to elicit test results that are directly proportional to the concentration of analyte in the sample within a given range. It should be established across the range of the analytical procedure. Linearity is usually expressed in terms of the variance around the slope of the regression line calculated according to an established mathematical relationship from test results obtained by the analysis of samples with varying concentrations of analyte, minimum of 6 concentrations.

The range of an analytical method is the interval between the upper and lower levels of analytics (including these levels) that have been determined with a suitable level of precision, accuracy, and linearity using the method as written. The range is normally expressed in the same unit as the test result (e.g. percent/ppm).

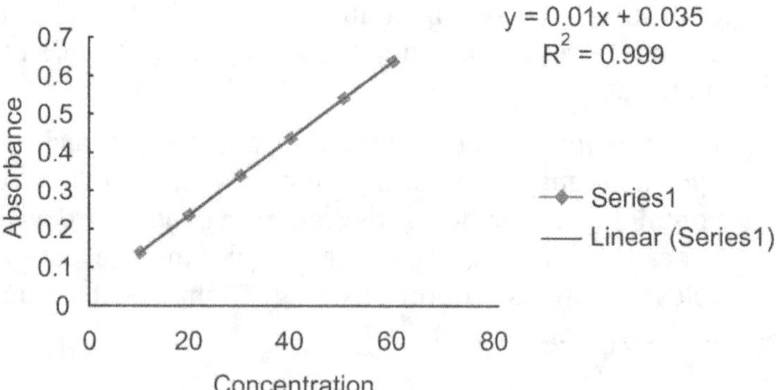

Fig. 12.2 Linearity and Range of API.

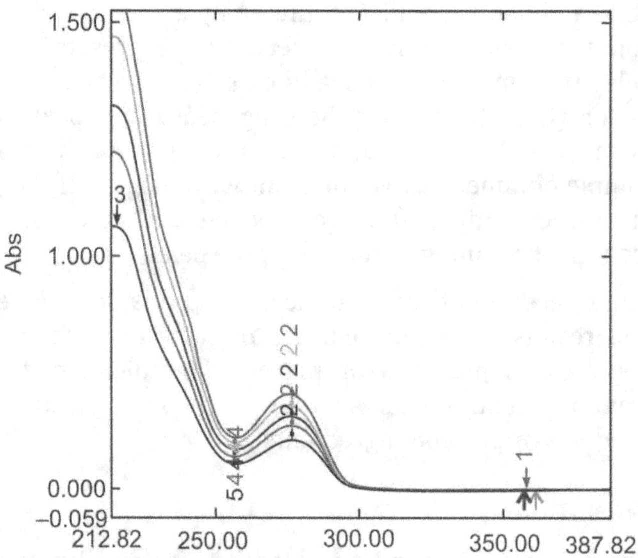

Fig. 12.3 Linearity and Range of API Spectra Overlay.

LIMIT OF DETECTION

Limit of detection (LOD) is the lowest amount of analyte in a sample that can be detected, but not necessarily quantitative, under the stated experimental conditions. The detection limits are usually expressed as the concentration of analyte (e.g., percentage ppb) in the sample.

> Expressed as a concentration at a specified signal: noise ratio.

> Determination based on

- Visual evaluation (non-instrumental and instrumental methods)
- Signal to noise (baseline noise)
- The standard deviation of response (s) and slope (S)

DL=3.3s/S, Estimation of S, from the calibration curve of the analyte.

Estimation of s, from the standard deviation of the blank, from the standard deviation (regression line or y-intercept) of a calibration curve in the range of the DL.

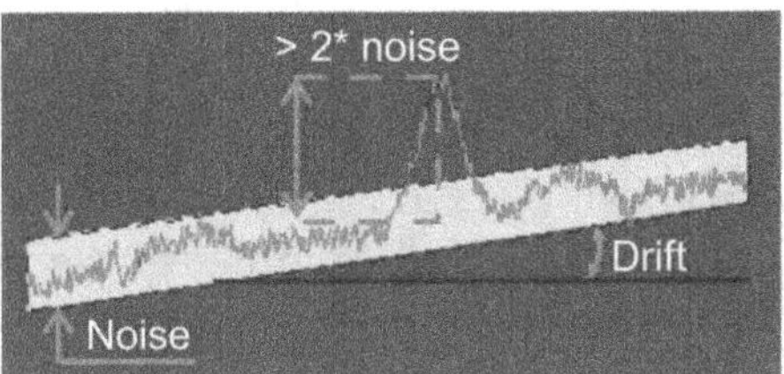

Fig.12.4 For Limit of detection shows noise by zooming baseline.

LIMIT OF QUANTITATION

The limit of quantitation (LOQ) is the lowest amount of analyte in a sample that can be determined with acceptable precision and accuracy under the stated experimental conditions. It is expressed as the concentration of analyte (e.g., percentage, ppb) in the sample.

> Determination based on

- Visual evaluation (non-instrumental and instrumental methods)
- Signal to noise (baseline noise)
- The standard deviation of response (s) and slope (S)

QL=10s/S, Estimation of S, from the calibration curve of the analyte.

Estimation of s, from the standard deviation of the blank, from the standard deviation (regression line or y-intercept) of a calibration curve in the range of the QL.

RUGGEDNESS

The ruggedness of an analytical method is the degree of reproducibility of test results obtained by the analysis of the same samples under a variety of conditions, such as different laboratories, different analysts, different instruments, different lots of reagents, different elapsed assay times, different assay temperature, different days, etc. Ruggedness is normally expressed as the lack of influence on test results of the operational and environmental variables of the analytical method.

ROBUSTNESS

The robustness of the analytical method is a measure of its capacity to remain unaffected by small but deliberate variations in method parameters and indicates its reliability during normal usage. A good practice is to vary important parameters in the method systematically and measure their effect on separation. Such parameters include mobile phase composition and pH, mobile phase additives, column temperature, flow rate etc.

STABILITY

The stability of sample, standard and reagents used in HPLC and UV method is required for a reasonable time to generate reproducible and reliable results. For example, 24-hour stability is desired for solutions and reagents that must be prepared for each analysis. Long term column stability is critical for method ruggedness since even the best HPLC column will eventually degrade and loose its initial performance.

Solutes may readily decompose prior to chromatographic investigations, e.g. during sample preparation, extraction, cleanup, phase transfer or storage of prepared vials (refrigerators or automatic sampler). Method development should investigate the stability of the analytes&standards.

System stability

- Stability of the samples being analyzed in a sample solution.
- The measure of the bias in assay results generated during a preselected time interval, e.g. 1 – 48 hours using a single solution
- Should be determined by replicate analysis of the sample solution.

- Considered appropriate when the RSD, calculated on the assay results obtained at different time intervals, is Less than 20 percent of the corresponding value of the system precision.

SYSTEM SUITABILITY TESTS

System suitability tests ensure that the method developed can generate acceptable accuracy and precision results. The USP defines parameters that can be used to determine system suitability prior to analysis. These parameters include column efficiency (N), peak asymmetry factor (As), resolution (Rs), capacity factor (k') and/or separation factor (α) and relative standard deviation (RSD) of peak area.

➢ Before or during analysis of unknowns, the checking of a system to ensure system performance.

➢ "No sample analysis is acceptable unless the requirements for system suitability have been met." *(USP Chapter 621)*

- Plate Count, Tailing, Resolution
- Determination of reproducibility (%RSD)

➢ For %RSD < 2.0%, Five replicates

➢ For %RSD > 2.0%, Six replicates

➢ System Suitability "Sample "- A mixture of main components and expected by-products utilized to determine system suitability

➢ "Whenever there is a significant change in equipment or reagents system suitability testing should be performed" (USP Chapter 621)

THIRTEEN

APPLICATIONS OF COLUMN CHROMATOGRAPY AND HPLC

- Column Chromatography is used to isolate active ingredients.
- It is very helpful in Separating compound mixtures.
- It is used to determine drug estimation from drug formulations
- It is used to remove impurities.
- Used to isolate metabolites from biological fluids.
- The main advantage of this chromatography technique is that the stationary phase is less expensive and can be easily disposed of as it undergoes recycling.
- Non-polar compounds. The polar compounds will strongly commune with the silica when compared to the non-polar compounds.
- Separation • purification • Isolation of active constituents • clinical

PHARMACEUTICAL SECTOR

- To identify and analyze samples for the presence of trace elements or chemicals.
- Separation of compounds based on their molecular weight and element composition.
- Detects the unknown compounds and purity of mixture.
- In drug development.

CHEMICAL INDUSTRY

- In testing water samples and also checks air quality.
- HPLC and GC are very much used for detecting various contaminants such as polychlorinated biphenyl (PCBs) in pesticides and oils.
- In various life sciences applications

FOOD INDUSTRY

- In food spoilage and additive detection
- Determining the nutritional quality of food

FORENSIC SCIENCE

- Forensic pathology and crime scene testing like analyzing blood and hair samples of crime places.

MOLECULAR BIOLOGY STUDIES

- Various hyphenated techniques in chromatography, such as EC-LC-MS, are applied in the study of metabolomics and proteomics along with nucleic acid research.
- HPLC is used in Protein Separation like Insulin Purification, Plasma Fractionation, and Enzyme Purification and also in various departments like Fuel Industry, biotechnology, and biochemical processes.

Separation of a mixture of compounds

- ➤ Purification process
- ➤ Isolation of active constituents
- ➤ Estimation of drugs in formulation
- ➤ Isolation of active constituents
- ➤ Determination of primary and secondary glycosides in digitalis leaf.
- ➤ Separation of diastereomers.

APPLICATIONS OF HPLC

The information that can be obtained by HPLC includes resolution, identification and quantification of a compound. It also aids in chemical separation and purification. The other applications of HPLC include:

- **Pharmaceutical Applications**
    1. To control drug stability.
    2. Tablet dissolution study of the pharmaceutical dosage form.
    3. Pharmaceutical quality control.
- **Environmental Applications**
    1. Detection of phenolic compounds in drinking water.
    2. Bio-monitoring of pollutants.
- **Applications in Forensics**
    1. Quantification of drugs in biological samples.
    2. Identification of steroids in blood, urine etc.
    3. Forensic analysis of textile dyes.
    4. Determination of cocaine and other drugs of abuse in blood, urine etc.
- **Food and Flavour**
    1. Measurement of Quality of soft drinks and water.
    2. Sugar analysis in fruit juices.
    3. Analysis of polycyclic compounds in vegetables.
    4. Preservative analysis.
- **Applications in Clinical Tests**
    1. Urine analysis, antibiotics analysis in blood.
    2. Analysis of bilirubin, biliverdin in hepatic disorders.
    3. Detection of endogenous Neuropeptides in the extracellular fluid of the brain etc.

PHARMACEUTICAL INDUSTRY

With the widespread production of pharmaceuticals came the legislation to ensure proper production and purity of drugs distributed. HPLC is among the most commonly used methods to verify drug purity globally.

Its use in assessing drugs on an industrial scale started in the 1980s, though its use in some countries is prevalent but still less widespread.

This can potentially be due to cost. HPLC is capable of providing sufficient precision for the industry standard, but only when it is preceded by calibration tests. This can increase the costs, but this sacrifice leads to high accuracy and specificity.

This means HPLC can be more beneficial in ensuring purity than other methods. The multiple crystallization method was previously used but had the drawback of potentially wasting expensive drugs. HPLC is much more efficient, and it minimizes losses to pharmaceutical manufacturers.

Even at the start of HPLC usage in the pharmaceutical industry, the method showed its usefulness. HPLC was used in the analysis of alkaloids, antibiotics, and steroids.

Steroids, in particular, were previously somewhat difficult to analyze owing to low dosages in medicines and the impractical forms they often came in (creams and ointments).

The early discussion focused on the detector used, a debate which still continues and evolves, but given the multitude of methods currently available, the debate is much more complex than it once was and can vary depending on the type of HPLC being considered.

HPLC is not only used for the analysis of finished drug products. Since HPLC can separate compounds, it is also applied during manufacture.

Through this separation, HPLC can provide critical starting products for the manufacture of new drugs or characterization of molecules with the potential to be manufactured into drugs.

These lead compounds can be derived from plants, animals, or fungi. HPLC can be used to separate enantiomers, the molecules that mirror images of each other, using chiral stationary phases (CSPs).

The ability to prove the purity of enantiomeric molecules is a standard in pharmaceutical assays, for which HPLC is suitable.

The most popular CSPs in pharmaceutical chemistry are polysaccharide benzoate and phenyl carbamate derivatives.

CLINICAL DIAGNOSIS

Catecholamines such as epinephrine and dopamine are highly important for many biological functions. Analyzing their precursors and metabolites can provide a diagnosis of diseases such as Parkinson's disease, heart disease, and muscular dystrophy.

However, given how physiologically widespread these molecules are, their analysis and subsequent conclusions about patient health must be done carefully. HPLC has the ability to separate and compare molecules to a higher magnitude than other techniques, making it a great candidate for such diagnostic purposes.

Reversed-phase HPLC (RP-HPLC) is one of the more popular methods due to its speed, column stability, and capacity to separate a wide range of compounds.

Identification of molecules in HPLC is made by measuring retention time. Retention time is the time it takes a molecule to pass through a column lined with adsorbents which interact differently with different molecules. This is done under varying conditions. In 1976, the potential use for RP-HPLC in diagnostic settings was shown.

Researchers exploited hydrophobic properties to separate catecholamine metabolites and amines in the same run, thereby speeding up the process. This is partly due to an interaction with pH, as acidic catecholamine metabolites are retained for longer at low pH values, but vice versa for amines.

Several conditions and settings can be modified in HPLC protocols. HPLC can then be used not only to detect diseases, as mentioned but also to monitor the progression of diseases.

Pheochromocytoma is a potentially fatal tumour of the sympathetic nervous system. It is derived from tissue in the neural crest, which implies that it secretes catecholamines. It can cause hypertension, which can complicate diagnosis, because it may only differ from hypertension in the format of its metabolites.

This makes HPLC ideal for diagnosis; however, the origin of the sample to be analyzed can affect the results. Urinary samples will reflect metabolites from both the central nervous system and the periphery.

Using cerebrospinal fluid offers results more localized to the central nervous system and is therefore preferred.

Table 13.1 Difference between Conventional chromatography and HPLC.

S.NO.	Conventional Chromatography	HPLC
1.	Plastic or glass columns used	Stainless steel columns used
2.	Generally, the length of columns10-100 cms	Generally, the length of columns is 10-30 cms
3.	Low resolution than HPLC	Higher resolution than other conventional chromatography
4.	Low-pressure sampling	High-pressure sampling
5.	Slower process than HPLC	Faster process than other conventional chromatography

HPLC finds its lot of applications not only confined to the isolation of natural pharmaceutically active compounds, control of micro-biological processes but also assay of pure drugs and their dosage forms. A few typical examples will be discussed below :

ISOLATION OF NATURAL PHARMACEUTICALLY ACTIVE COMPOUNDS

Some plant alkaloids and glycosides can be isolated as stated below :

Category of Medicinal Plant contains, for, e.g.

1. Glycoside contains in Digitalis & Sennosides used in Cardiovascular diseases & Laxatives,

2. Alkaloids such as Morphine & Codeine having Analgesic & Antitussive.

By HPLC, we can separate and find out Digitalis as per below using

Chromatographic Conditions:

Column   :   Size-25 cm × 4.6 mm ID ;

Adsorbent   :   Lichrosorb RP-8 ;

Mobile-phase :   Water/Acetonitrile-Gradient Elution ;

Detector   :   UV 254 nm

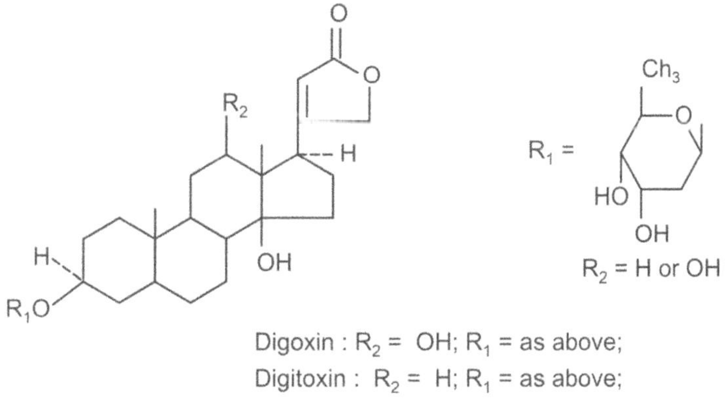

Fig. 13.1 Structure of Digoxin.

CONTROL OF MICROBIOLOGICAL PROCESSES

Various microbiological processes are used in the production of a number of antibiotics, for instance :

penicillins, tetracyclines, chloramphenicol and **streptomycins.**
The major areas of such operations being:

- kinetics of the microbiological process,

- monitoring of the ongoing process,

- isolation and purification of active ingredients,

- purity control of active constituents, and

- monitoring derivatization reactions of these compounds.

HPLC-controlled analysis of a microbiological process during Penicillin production: Chromatographic conditions are as follows :

Column   :   Size-25 cm × 4.6 mm ID ;

Adsorbent   : Lichrosorb-$NH_2^{(R)}$ (10 μ m) ;

Mobile-phase   :   0.005 M H_2SO_4 buffer (pH 4.4))/acetonitrile (50 : 50) ; Flow rate : 3 ml min^{-1} ;

Detector   :   UV-220 nm ;

Microbial cleavage of Penicillin-G into 6-AMP and phenylacetate is as shown below :

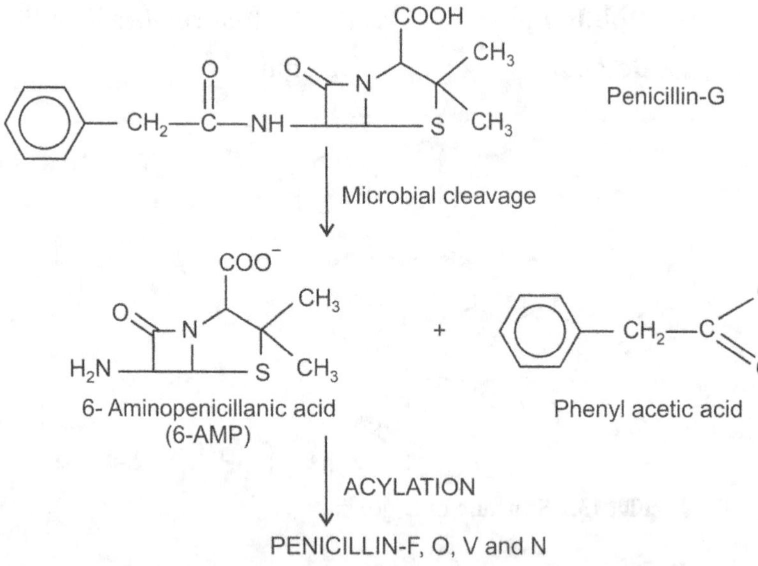

Fig. 13.2 Structure of Penicillin.

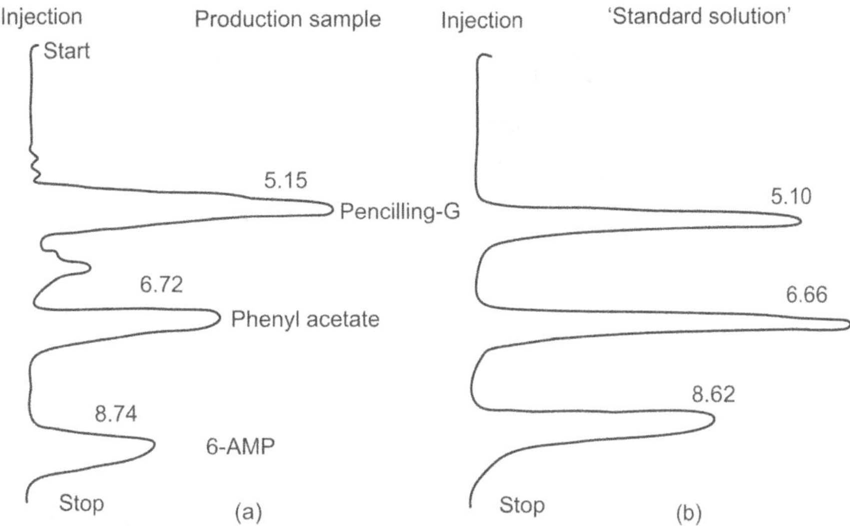

(a) and (b): HPLC Chromatograms of Penicillins In 'Production sample' and 'Standard solution'.

Fig. 13.3 HPLC Chromatogram of STD and Sample Penicillin.

The application of HPLC depended on the type of compounds and choice of Stationary phase and Mobile phase as follows, shown in the table below.

Table 13.2 Modes of Elution as per S.P & MP.

Types of compounds	Mode	Stationary Phase	Mobile Phase
Neutrals Weak Acids Weak Bases	Reversed Phase	C18, C8, C4 Cyano, amino	Water/Organic Modifiers
Ionics, Bases, Acids	Ion Pair	C-18, C-8	Water/Organic Ion-Pair Reagent
Compounds not soluble in water	Normal Phase	Silica, Amino, Cyno, Diol	Organics
Ionics Inorganic Ions	Ion Exchange	Anion or Cation Exchange Resin	Aqueous/Buffer Counter Ion
High Molecular Weight Compounds Polymer	Size Exclusion	Polystyrene Silica	Gel Filtration-Aqueous Gel Permeation-Organic

The following compounds can be separated by HPLC:

Bioscience

Proteins, peptides, nucleotides

Consumer Products

Lipids, antioxidants, sugars

Clinical

amino acids, vitamins, homocysteine

Pharmaceuticals

tetracyclines, corticosteroids, antidepressants, barbiturates

Environmental

polyaromatic hydrocarbons, Inorganic ions, herbicides

Chemical

Polystyrenes, dyes, phthalates

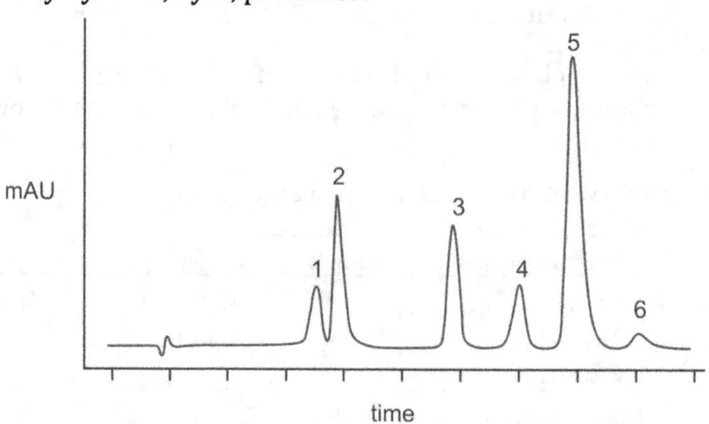

Fig. 13.4 HPLC Chromatogram of separation of Carbohydrate Sample.

The mixture of Carbohydrates separated as shown in above fig.no.13.4.

1. fructose

2. Glucose

3. Saccharose

4. Palatinose

5. Trehalulose

6. isomaltose

FOURTEEN

ULTRA HIGH-PERFORMANCE LIQUID CHROMATOGRAPHY (UPLC) OR (UHPLC)

INTRODUCTION

In 2004, separation science was revolutionized with the introduction of Ultra-Performance Liquid Chromatography [UPLC® Technology]. Significant advances in instrumentation and column technology were made to achieve dramatic increases in resolution, speed and sensitivity in liquid chromatography. For the first time, a holistic approach involving simultaneous innovations in particle technology and instrument design was modified to meet and overcome the challenges of the analytical laboratory. This was done in order to make analytical scientists more successful and businesses more profitable and productive.

For more than four decades, reducing stationary-phase particle size has been exploited to improve chromatographic separation efficiency. Until recently, LC technology had reached a plateau in which the benefits of reducing particle size could not be fully realized due to the negative influence of instrument band spreading and limited pressure range.

UPLC System has removed those barriers, enabling columns packed with smaller particles [1.7 – 1.8 µm] to reach their theoretical performance while precisely delivering mobile phase at pressures up to 1030 bar [15,000 psi], thus providing a high level of chromatographic performance.

UPLC Technology facilitates improvements in resolution, sensitivity, and speed to be achieved without compromise. Whether the separation goal is to achieve ultra-fast analysis, increase throughput while maintaining resolution, improving resolution while decreasing analysis time or achieve ultra-high resolution

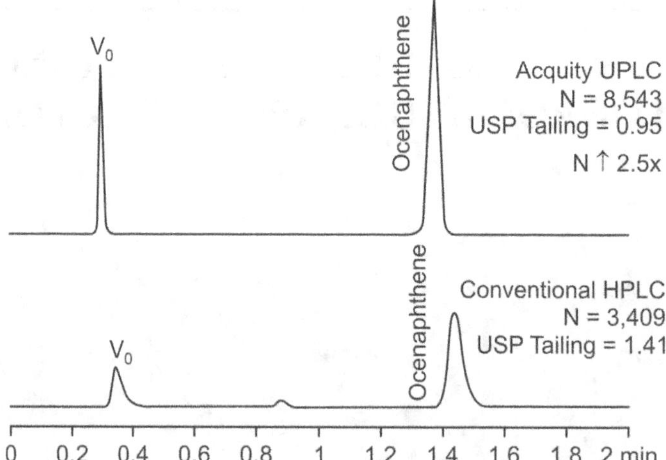

Fig. 14.1 UPLC & HPLC Chromatogram of separation of Ocenaphthene Sample.

- UPLC refers to ultra high-performance liquid chromatography.
- It improves chromatographic resolution, speed, and sensitivity in three areas.
- UHPLC is a rising chromatographic separation technique whose packing materials have smaller particular sizes lesser than 2.5µm.
- The technology takes full advantage of chromatographic principles to run separation using a column packed with smaller particles and higher flow rates

It can withstand high system back-pressure.

- Special analytical columns UHPLC BEH C18 packed with
- The factor responsible for the development of the UHPLC technique was the evolution of the packing material used to effect the separation.
- The technology takes full advantage of chromatographic principles to run separations using columns packed with smaller particles.
- It decreases analysis time and solvent consumption 1.7µm particles are used in connection with the system.

PRINCIPLE

The Principle of UHPLC is based on the Van Deemeter equation, which describes the relationship between flow rate and HETP or column efficiency. H=A + B/v + Cv when, A= Eddy diffusion B= Longitudinal diffusion C= equilibrium mass transfer v= flow rate Van Deemeter equation that describes the relationship between linear velocity (flow rate) and plate height (HETP or column efficiency) as disused in HPLC.

COMPARISON BETWEEN HPLC AND UHPLC

Parameters HPLC

Column Type C_{18}, 50 × 4.6mm

Flow rate 5.0 ml per min 01.0 ml per min

Injection volume 100 µl 20 µl partial loop fill or 50 µl full loop fill

Total run time 30 min 5 mins

Theoretical Plate count is 2000 to 10000.

Pressure applied 500-5000 Psi

Parameters UHPLC

AQUITY UHPLC BEH C_{18},50 ×2.1mm Particle size 4µm particles 1.7µm particles

Flow rate 3.0 ml per min 0.6 ml per min

Injection volume 20 µl 3 µl partial loop fill or 5 µl full loop fill

Total run time 10 min 1.5 min

Theoretical Plate count 10000 to 20000

Pressure applied 2000-20000 Psi

UHPLC Lower limit of quantization 0.2 µg/ml 0.054µl/ml

A completely new system design with advanced technology in the pump, autosampler, detector, data system, and service diagnostics was required.

- The ACQUITY UHPLC system has been designed for low system and dwells volume.
- Achieving small particle, high peak capacity separations require a greater pressure range than that achievable by the HPLC system.

INSTRUMENTATION

1. **SOLVENT RESERVOIR:** Most manufacturers supply these bottles with special caps, tubing and filters to connect to the pump inlet, and so the purge gas (helium) is used to remove dissolved air. The most common type of solvent reservoir is a glass bottle.

2. **PUMPS USED IN UHPLC:** Same as used in HPLC previously discussed in detail.

RECIPROCATING PISTON PUMP: Same used in HPLC with High Pressure.

Reciprocating piston pumps:

- Consists of a small motor-driven piston which moves rapidly back and front in a hydraulic chamber that may vary from 35-400µl in volume.

- On the backstroke, the separation column valve is closed, and the piston pulls insolvent from the mobile phase reservoir.

- On the forward stroke, the pump pushes solvent out of the column from the reservoir.

Syringe type pump:

- These are most suitable for small bore columns because this pump delivers only a finite volume of mobile phase before it has to be refilled. These pumps have a volume between 250 to 500ml.

- The pump operates by a motorized lead screw that delivers the mobile phase to the column at a constant rate. The rate of solvent delivery is controlled by changing the voltage on the motor.

CONSTANT FLOW PUMP: This type is mostly used in all common UPLC application

Constant pressure pump

CONSTANT PRESSURE PUMP: Constant pressure is used only for column packing

- In these types of pumps, the mobile phase is driven through the column with the use of pressure from the gas cylinder.

- A low-pressure gas source is needed to generate high liquid pressure.

- The valving arrangement allows the rapid refill of the solvent chamber, whose capacity is about 70ml.

3. SAMPLE INJECTION:

- In UHPLC, a sample introduction is critical. Conventional injection valves, either automated or manual, and hardened to work at extreme pressure.

- To protect the column from extreme pressure fluctuations, the injection process must be relatively pulse-free, and the swept volume of the device also needs to be minimal to reduce potential band spreading.

- Low volume injections with minimal carryover are required to increase sensitivity.

4. UHPLC COLUMN:

The UHPLC column plays an important role in the resolution of the peak, as shown in fig no 14.2

- Resolution is increased in a 1.7μm particle packed column because it is better. •Separation of the components of a sample requires a bonded phase that provides both retention and selectivity. • Four bonded phases are available for UHPLC separations: ACQUITY UHPLC BEH C_{18} and C_8 (straight-chain alkyl columns), ACQUITY UHPLC BEH shield RP $_{18}$ (embedded polar group column), ACQUITY UHPLC BEH (phenyl group tethered to the silyl functionality with a C6 alkyl) ACQUITY UHPLC BEH Amide columns (trifunctionally bonded amide phase).

ACQUITY UHPLC BEH C_{18} and C_8:

- These are considered the universal columns of choice for most UHPLC separation by providing the widest pH range.
- The low pH stability is combined with the high pH stability of the 1.7μm BEH particle to deliver the widest unstable pH operating range. ACQUITY UHPLC BEH shield RP 18: These are designed to provide selectivity that complements the ACQUITY UPLC BEH T M C_{18} and C_8 columns.

  BEH amide columns facilities the use of a wide range of phase pH

  o BEH particle technology, in combination with a trifunctionally bonded amide phase, provides exceptional column lifetime, thus improving assay robustness.

  o ACQUITY UHPLC BEH phenyl columns: These utilize trifunctional C6 alkyl ethyl between the phenyl ring. Enhanced mechanical stability bridging the methyl group in the silica matrix.

- ACQUITY UHPLC BEH AMIDE COLUMNS:

CHEMISTRY OF SMALL PARTICLES

- As the particle size decreases to less than 2.5μm, not only there is a significant gain in efficiency, but the efficiency doesn't diminish at increased flow rates.

- By using smaller particles, speed and peak capacity (number of peaks resolved per unit time in gradient separation) can be extended to new limits, termed ultra-performance liquid chromatography.

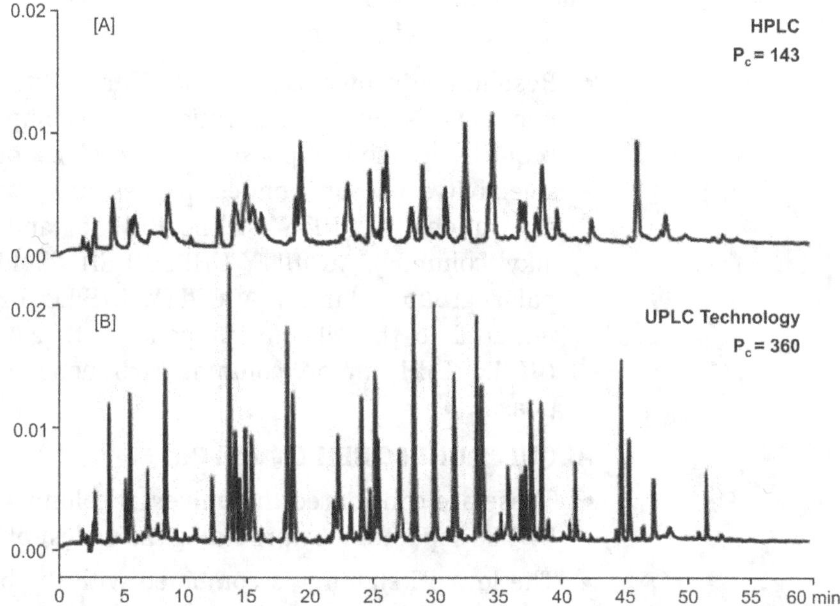

Fig. 14.2 UPLC & HPLC Chromatogram of separation of Complex Sample.

DETECTORS

- UV Detectors
- Fluorescent detector
- Refractive index detector
- Light scattering detector
- Electrochemical detector
- Mass spectrometric detector.

PHOTOTUBE

- Consist of high sensitive cathode in a form of half cylinder in evacuated tube.
- Anode is also present along the axis of the tube.
- Inside layer is coated with light sensitive layer.
- When light is incident, surface coating emits electron this is attracted and collected by anode.

- Current which is created between cathode and anode is regarded as measure of radiation falling On the detector.

PHOTOMULTIPLIER TUBE

Ejected photoelectron strikes dynode secondary electron released voltage accelerates electron to next dynode Result is large charge packet hitting anode High gain and detected.

FLUORESCENCE DETECTOR

- The light from an excitation source passes through a filter or monochromator and strikes the sample.
- A proportion of the incident light is absorbed by the sample and some of the molecules in the sample fluorescence. The fluorescent light is emitted in all directions.
- Some of this fluorescent light passes through a second filter or monochromator and reaches a detector, which is usually placed at 90° to the incident light beam to minimize the risk of transmitted or reflected incident light reaching the detector.

REFRACTIVE INDEX DETECTOR

- This detector based on the deflection principle of refractory, where the deflection of a light beam is changed when the composition in the sample flow cell changes in relation to the reference side.
- As sample elutes through one side, the changing angle of refraction moves the beam.
- This result in a change in the photon current falling on the detector which unbalances it. The extent of unbalance is recorded on a strip chart recorder.

ADVANTAGES OF UHPLC

- Decreases run time and increases sensitivity.
- Reducing analysis time so that more product can be produced with existing resources.
- Provides the selectivity, sensitivity and dynamic range of LC analysis
- Maintains resolution performance
- Fast resolving power quickly quantifies related and unrelated compounds.

- Operation cost is reduced.
- Less solvent consumption.

DISADVANTAGES OF UHPLC

- Due to increased pressure requires more maintenance and reduces the life of the columns of this type.
- In addition, the phases of less than 2μm are generally non-regenerable and thus have limited use.

APPLICATION OF UHPLC

- Analysis of natural products and traditional herbal medicine.
- Identification of metabolite
- Study of metabonomics/metablomics
- Bio analysis/bioequivalence studies.
- Manufacturing/QA/QC
- Impurity profiling
- Forced degradation studies
- Dissolution testing
- Toxicity studies.

It provides high speed, accuracy and reproducible results for analysis of drugs and their related substance. Thus method development time decrease.

- UPLC used for accurate, reliable and reproducible analysis of amino acids in area of protein characterization, cell culture monitoring and nutritional analysis of food.

5. DETECTORS:

UV Detectors
- Fluorescent detector
- Refractive index detector
- Light scattering detector
- Electrochemical detector
- Mass spectrometric detector.

PHOTOTUBE:

- It consists of a highly sensitive cathode in the form of a half-cylinder in an evacuated tube.
- Anode is also present along the axis of the tube.

- Inside layer is coated with light-sensitive layer.
- When light is incident, surface coating emits an electron; this is attracted and collected by the anode.
- Current, which is created between cathode and anode, is regarded as a measure of radiation falling on the detector.

PHOTOMULTIPLIER TUBE

Ejected photoelectron strikes dynode secondary electron released voltage accelerates electron to next dynode Result is large charge packet hitting anode High gain and detected.

FLUORESCENCE DETECTOR

- The light from an excitation source passes through a filter or monochromator and strikes the sample.
- A proportion of the incident light is absorbed by the sample and some of the molecules in the sample fluorescence. The fluorescent light is emitted in all directions.
- Some of this fluorescent light passes through a second filter or monochromator and reaches a detector, which is usually placed at 90° to the incident light beam to minimize the risk of transmitted or reflected incident light reaching the detector.

REFRACTIVE INDEX DETECTOR

- This detector is based on the deflection principle of refractory, where the deflection of a light beam is changed when the composition in the sample flow cell changes in relation to the reference side.
- As the sample elutes through one side, the changing angle of refraction moves the beam.
- This results in a change in the photon current falling on the detector, which unbalances it. The extent of unbalance is recorded on a strip chart recorder.

ADVANTAGES OF UHPLC

- Decreases run time and increases sensitivity.
- Reducing analysis time so that more product can be produced with existing resources.

- Provides the selectivity, sensitivity and dynamic range of LC analysis
- Maintains resolution performance
- Fast resolving power quickly quantifies related and unrelated compounds.
- Operation cost is reduced.
- Less solvent consumption.

DISADVANTAGES OF UHPLC

- Due to increased pressure requires more maintenance and reduces the life of the columns of this type.
- In addition, the phases of less than 2µm are generally non-regenerable and thus have limited use.

APPLICATION OF UHPLC

- Analysis of natural products and traditional herbal medicine.
- Identification of metabolite
- Study of metabonomics/metablomics
- Bioanalysis/bioequivalence studies.
- Manufacturing/QA/QC
- Impurity profiling
- Forced degradation studies
- Dissolution testing
- Toxicity studies.

It provides high speed, accuracy and reproducible results for the analysis of drugs and their related substance. Thus method development time decrease.

- UPLC is used for accurate, reliable and reproducible analysis of amino acids in the area of protein characterization, cell culture monitoring and nutritional analysis of food.